CW01496698

PRIMAL

FASTING

BUILD HEALTH AND STRENGTH

WITH

TIME-RESTRICTED FEEDING

AND

PROGRESSIVE RESISTANCE TRAINING

Don Matesz, M.A., M.S., L.Ac.

Primal Fasting

Don Matesz, M.A., M.S., L.Ac.

INTEGRITY PRESS

2018

Primal Fasting

First Edition

Copyright © 2018 Donald A. Matesz

All rights reserved

ISBN-13: 978-1979527514

ISBN-10: 1979527512

Front cover photo © Andrey Kuzmin/Shutterstock
License

No part of this book may be reproduced or transmitted
in any form or by any means, electronic or mechanical,
including photocopying, recording, or by any
information storage and retrieval system, except for
brief excerpts for the purposes of review and
commentary, without written permission from the
copyright holder.

CONTENTS

Note To The Reader

Diet has a powerful effect on health and fitness. If you are seriously ill or on medications, consult a health care provider knowledgable about nutrition and its health effects and about your medications before you make any changes to your diet or exercise program. You remain always responsible for your choices, actions, and their consequences. This book serves as educational information only and does not substitute for the guidance of a health care professional familiar with your unique situation. Nothing herein is to be construed as a diagnosis or treatment plan for any individual's unique physical condition.

1 Why Fast?

Everyone goes without eating some part of every day, and we know that people living previous to the modern industrial age fasted for longer periods of time and more often than most people do today. From time immemorial people have used fasting as a means to improve physical health and advance spiritual development.

Due to daily and seasonal fluctuations in wild food supplies, as well as absence of artificial lighting, many mammals, including anthropoid apes and preagricultural humans, eat less often and fast more frequently than modern people and domesticated animals. This is especially true of large carnivores; a wild wolf or lion might eat only once every few days, depending on seasonal opportunity to capture game. Mammals including humans have specific metabolic adaptations to regularly going extended periods without food:

> "The ability to function at a high level, both physically and mentally, during extended periods

without food may have been of fundamental importance in our evolutionary history. Many adaptations to periodic reductions of food supply are conserved among mammals, including organs for the uptake and storage of rapidly mobilizable glucose (liver glycogen stores) and longer-lasting energy substrates, such as fatty acids in adipose tissue."[1]

A growing body of evidence indicates that frequent feeding is discordant with our biology, contributing to the development of disorders such as obesity, metabolic syndrome and non-insulin dependent diabetes mellitus. These disorders represent the body's attempt to cope with too frequent and excess food intake.

---

1 Mattson MP, Allison DB, Fontana L, et al., "Meal frequency and timing in health and disease," Proceedings of the National Academy of Sciences of the United States of America. 2014;111(47):16647-16653. <http://www.ncbi.nlm.nih.gov/pmc/articles/PMC4250148/>

Our hunter-gatherer ancestors had less famine than modern farmers,[2] but their food intake fluctuated more on a regular basis. Because they did not have refrigerators or restaurants, our hunting ancestors could not always eat three meals daily.

Contemporary hunter-gatherers generally spent their mornings and early afternoons foraging for foods. Before or during hunting or foraging, a hunter-gatherer might eat some leftovers, dried meat, nuts, seeds or berries found along the way. After obtaining food, they trekked back to home base to prepare the day's one large main meal. This means that a hunter-gatherer either fasted completely, or had very little to eat during 16-20 of the 24 hours daily. Today we call this *time-restricted feeding* (TRF) and *intermittent energy restriction* (IER).

In addition, at least several times a month they'd have to go a day or two with very little or nothing to eat when unable to garner game or procure plants due to

---

[2] Berbesque JC, Marlowe FW, Shaw P, Thompson P. Hunter–gatherers have less famine than agriculturalists. *Biology Letters*. 2014;10(1):20130853. doi:10.1098/rsbl.2013.0853. <https://www.ncbi.nlm.nih.gov/pmc/articles/PMC3917328/>

fluctuations in animal activity and plant growth. Today this is called *intermittent fasting* (IF).

Those human ancestors who had plenty of energy for gathering food during a prolonged daily or weekly fast of this sort thrived and left more children than those who couldn't move unless they had food in their stomachs. You inherited that ability from those people who were well-adapted to being active on an empty stomach (those who didn't thrive when fasted didn't have descendants leading to you).

Among traditional horticulturalists and agriculturalists, adults didn't eat much if anything until after spending several hours in the morning and/or before noon doing farm or kitchen chores (including preparing the first meal from scratch). The English word "dinner" comes from the Old French *disner* which originally meant "breakfast," that is, the meal that comes after the extended daily fast. In French and English "dinner" traditionally referred to the main meal of the day, which in pre-industrial times was taken sometime between late morning and midday (after morning work). The second, smaller meal was supper, usually taken well before sunset. The word "lunch" originally meant "hunk of bread"[3] and referred to an afternoon snack – not a full meal – had between the first (midday) meal and supper. Only the wealthy, overfed aristocrats ate more than two main meals daily, and they were most prone to obesity, gout, and other diseases.

Ancient people placed great importance on fasting as a means of arousing dreams, visions, or ecstasy. Our ancient hunter-gatherer ancestors practiced shamanic religion to explore human awareness and spiritual potential. In shamanic cultures, shamans and in many cases youths on the verge of adulthood practiced fasting as preparation for their interior journeys to the spirit world to obtain guidance through visions.[4]

Most agricultural religions – including Jainism, Buddhism, Daoism (a.k.a. Taoism), Hinduism, and the Abrahamic traditions – incorporate some form or

---

[3] According to the Oxford English Dictionary, the word "bread" originally meant "piece of food" and is related to "break (into pieces)." Also, the Old English word "bræd" meant "flesh." Hence "bread" did not originally refer only to the grain flour product, which explains why the word "sweetbread" refers to the pancreas of an animal used as food.

[4] Harner M, *The Way of the Shaman* (HarperOne, 1990).

degree of fasting as a method of spiritual expression or development.

In ancient Greece, it was believed that eating risked entry of demonic beings that caused disease and shortened life.[5] As in shamanic cultures, among the Greeks fasting was required to prepare for many rituals by which someone sought guidance from spiritual entities. Pythagoras, Abaris, and Epimenides all recommended fasting.

Buddhism is an ancient religion. In the Kitagiri Sutta of the Majjhima Nikaya, Gautama the Buddha is depicted as recommending that his followers restrict themselves to two meals daily, taken in morning and at mid-day – *time-restricted feeding* – as a method for establishing good health:

> "I, monks, abstain from the night-time meal. As I abstain from the night-time meal, I sense next-to-no illness, next-to-no affliction, lightness,

---

[5] Kerndt PR, Naughton JL, Driscoll CE, Loxterkamp DA, "Fasting: The History, Pathophysiology and Complications," *Western Journal of Medicine*. 1982;137(5):379-399.
<http://www.ncbi.nlm.nih.gov/pmc/articles/PMC1274154/?page=3>

strength, and a comfortable abiding. Come now. You too abstain from the night-time meal. As you are abstaining from the night-time meal, you, too, will sense next-to-no illness, next-to-no affliction, lightness, strength, and a comfortable abiding."[6]

According to some legends, Bodhidharma, a patriarch of Chinese chán (zen) Buddhism, practiced limited fasting during his quest for spiritual awakening.[7]

Similar to the Greeks, ancient (and some modern) Daoists believed that eating grains (Pinyin: *gu*) or any excess food feeds three worms that cause all diseases. An ancient Daoist text called "Writings of the Masters of Huainan" asserts:

"Those who eat meat are brave but cruel.
Those who eat Qi have bright spirits and long lives.
Those who eat grains are intelligent but die early.
Those who do not eat at all are immortal."

---

[6] Kitagiri Sutta: At Kitagiri. Trans. by Thanissaro Bhikkhu, 2005. <http://www.accesstoinsight.org/tipitaka/mn/mn.070.than.html>

[7] Eisen M, "Chinese Bigu for Yang Sheng," *Yang Sheng* 2011 October 15. <http://yang-sheng.com/?p=3874>

Apparently these Daoists had some idea that fasting promoted longevity. Since at least 200 B.C., Daoists have practiced *bigu* – fasting and food restriction, particularly grain (Pinyin: *gu*) avoidance – as a means of health and spiritual cultivation and to develop immortality.[8] Some ancient Chinese artists practiced fasting to purify their minds and grasp a vision for their artistic expression.

Similar to shamanic cultures, in the Biblical Old and New Testament, fasting was regarded as a powerful preparation for divine revelations. The New Testament depicts Jesus undertaking a 40 day fast in the desert, during which he has visions, obtains revelations, and develops his spiritual power. Similar stories appear in other traditions.

Many members of the modern Seventh-Day Adventist Christian sect follow the advice of the church's founder, Ellen White, to eat only two meals daily – morning and afternoon – and thus have longer daily

---

[8] Eisen M, "Chinese Bigu for Yang Sheng," *Yang Sheng* 2011 October 15. <http://yang-sheng.com/?p=3874>

fasts (16-18 hours). Members of the modern Church of Latter Day Saints (Mormons) are encouraged to do an absolute fast for 24 hours at least once monthly, starting from the age of 8 years old. Seventh-Day Adventists and Mormons who practice fasting appear to enjoy better health than those who do not, as discussed below.

Today we know that periods of complete fasting (no food at all) of sufficient duration elicit beneficial metabolic states in the brain and heart. These metabolic states may help an individual to elicit states of consciousness that contribute to artistic and spiritual insight and development.

In summary, it seems that in traditional (pre-industrial) cultures most people spent 16 to 20 hours daily in the fasted (yang) state and only 4 to 8 hours in the fed (yin) state whereas modern people spend more like 12 to 16 hours in the fed (yin) state, and only 8 to 12 hours in the fasted (yang) state. They considered fasting a reliable method for improving health, increasing lifespan and developing wisdom and spiritual power.

Modern people feed too often, and fast too little. This means they are full more often than they are empty. Eating too often and fasting too little inevitably results in accumulations of excess nutriment and waste in the body, which promotes disease. It may also make our minds dull, insensitive, and less capable of experiencing the full range of higher, insightful states of consciousness described by shamans and wisdom seekers throughout time.

2 Defining Primal Fasting

Historically the word "fasting" has referred to any voluntary reduction of or abstinence from some or all food or nutritive beverages for a period of time. An absolute fast consists of abstaining from all nutritive food and beverages other than water for a specific period of time.

Chronic calorie restriction (CR) is an example of limited fasting, in which one or more types of food are restricted on a continuous daily basis, resulting in a substantial (20-40%) reduction of energy (calorie) intake, but without a change in meal frequency (number and timing of daily meals). Popular examples include conventional dieting, and some types of religious fasting that restrict specific foods but not others, including the Biblical Daniel Fast and the Greek Orthodox fasting rituals (discussed below). The CR Society International promotes chronic calorie restriction with optimal nutrition (CRON) as a path to longevity.

Periodic or intermittent absolute fasting – also known as water fasting – involves incorporating into one's diet regular periods of 16-36 hours during which one does not consume any food or nutritive beverages. There exist two common strategies for intermittent fasting for health benefits. One involves fasting for about 24 hours once or twice weekly, perhaps occasionally for longer periods of time.

Another approach involves limiting daily intake of food and nutritive beverages to a specific time window – e.g. 1-8 hours - hence producing periods of absolute fasting for 16-23 hours daily. As already noted, this is sometimes called time-restricted feeding (TRF), and was the normal way of eating for non-agricultural people and most of humanity prior to the industrial age.

Some people use the term "intermittent fasting" to refer to both periodic absolute fasting and time-restricted feeding. The word "intermittent" may not be ideal because it means "occurring at irregular intervals." If people use absolute fasting and time-restricted feeding at more or less regular intervals such as once or twice weekly for absolute fasting and daily for time-restricted feeding, it may be more accurate to call this periodic fasting, since "periodic" means "recurring at intervals of time."

As noted, the CR Society International promotes chronic calorie-restriction with optimal nutrition (CRON) as a path to longevity. There exists considerable evidence that chronic caloric restriction delays aging and prolongs lifespan in non-primate animals. A 23-year study found that caloric restriction alone did reduce disease risks and reduce the rate of aging, but did not extend the lives of rhesus monkeys.[9]

The CR Society International warns that chronic caloric restriction may mean chronic hunger, preoccupation with food, physical wasting, loss of libido, and impaired fertility. Loss of libido leads to low procreative activity. Any ancient humans who deliberately restricted food intake when food was available would have had fewer offspring than those who ate to satisfaction whenever possible. Chronic caloric

---

[9] NIH. "Calorie Restriction May Not Extend Life," *NIH Research Matters* 2012 September 17. <https://www.nih.gov/news-events/nih-research-matters/calorie-restriction-may-not-extend-life>

restriction does not resonate with our evolved biology, what I call our True Nature.

As noted, fasting refers to any type of voluntary food restriction. For example, a vegetarian or vegan regimen restricting animal products is a type of fast: fasting from some or all animal products. Along this line, although not a common practice, we can also regard deliberate restriction of some or all plant foods as a type of fasting: fasting (abstaining) from carbohydrates.

As we go back in time, or examine wild foods, it appears clear that the natural and ancestral diet of man included much less carbohydrate (starch and sugar) than agricultural diets based on grains. Ancient Europeans ate highly carnivorous diets, similar to canine species like the fox and wolf.[10] The Roman historian Tacitus reported that the native Germans of Europe ate a diet of wild game, curdled milk products, and wild fruits, which supply little carbohydrate – in

[10] Richards MP. A brief review of the archaeological evidence for Palaeolithic and Neolithic subsistence. Eur J Clin Nutr. 2002 Dec;56(12): 16 p following 1262. PubMed PMID: 12494313.

short, a low carbohydrate diet.[11] Contemporary hunter-gatherer tribes ate animal-based diets without grains and relatively low in digestible carbohydrate.[12] As mentioned, ancient Daoists believed that eating starchy grains fed diseases and reduced lifespan. Modern science has provided some support for this view.

Some evidence suggests that the benefits of caloric restriction are due primarily to restriction of carbohydrate intake and consequent reduction of chronic insulin exposure. Glucose restriction (i.e. reduced carbohydrate metabolism) shifts cell metabolism to fatty acid oxidation, which increases mitochondrial respiration and oxidative stress, which in turn stimulates an increase in stress defense

[11] Tacitus. Germania and Agricola. Ostara Publications, 2016. Page 9. "Their food is of a simple kind, consisting of wild fruit, fresh game, and curdled milk." They used grains to make alcohol, which weakened them. "If you indulge their love of drinking by supplying them with as much as they desire, they will be overcome by their own vices as easily as by the arms of an enemy."

[12] Cordain L, Miller JB, Eaton SB, Mann N, Holt SH, Speth JD. Plant-animal subsistence ratios and macronutrient energy estimations in worldwide hunter-gatherer diets. Am J Clin Nutr. 2000 Mar;71(3):682-92. PubMed PMID:10702160.

responses with a marked increase in lifespan.[13, 14] On the other hand, glucose feeding increases insulin exposure and IGF-1 activity and shortens life span in worms and likely mammals because the insulin-signaling pathway is evolutionarily well conserved from worms to mammals.[15]

Humans have no dietary requirement for carbohydrate,[16] so dietary carbohydrate restriction is a rational type of food restriction – fasting – that enjoys

[13] Schulz T, Karse K, Voigt A, et al.. Glucose restriction extends Caenorhabditis elegans life span by inducing mitochondrial respiration and increasing oxidative stress. Cell Metabolism 2007 Oct 3;6(4):280-293. <http://www.sciencedirect.com/science/article/pii/S1550413107002562>

[14] Kenyon C, Chang J, Gensch E, et al. A C. elegans mutant that lives twice as lone as wild type. Nature 1993;366:461-464.

[15] Lee S, Murphy CT, Kenyon C. Glucose shortens the life span of C. elegans by downregulating DAF-16/FOXO activity and aquaporin gene expression. Cell metabolism 2009 Nov 4;10(5): 379-391.<http://www.sciencedirect.com/science/article/pii/S1550413109003027>

[16] Food and Nutrition Board, National Academy of Sciences. Dietary Reference Intakes for Energy, Carbohydrate, Fiber, Fat, Fatty Acids, Cholesterol, Protein, and Amino Acids. National Academies Press, 2005. Pages 275-6. "The lower limit of dietary carbohydrate compatible with life apparently is zero, provided that adequate amounts of protein and fat are consumed." <https://www.nap.edu/read/10490/chapter/8?term=carbohydrate+requirement#275>

scientific support and resonates with ancestral diets and the ancient Daoist practice of avoiding grains.

Some advocate protein restriction for reduction of excessive IGF-1 levels. Protein-restriction is unwise because protein is an essential nutrient and restriction is associated with adverse effects. Elderly people who eat diets low in animal protein have been found to have a significantly greater risk of bone loss and osteoporosis.[17] A low-carbohydrate, high protein diet slows tumor growth and prevents cancer initiation.[18]

In this booklet, you will learn the benefits of what I call primal fasting, because it mimics the fasting patterns of our ancestors: implementing daily time-restricted feeding, and either periodic or intermittent 20-24 hour absolute fasting, to enhance the benefits of a whole foods, meat-based, carbohydrate-restricted diet, which

---

[17] Hannan MT, Tucker KL, Dawson-Hughes B, et al. Effect of dietary protein on bone loss in elderly men and women: The Framingham Osteoporosis Study. J Bone Min Res 2000 Dec 1;15(12):2504-12. <http://onlinelibrary.wiley.com/doi/10.1359/jbmr.2000.15.12.2504/full>

[18] Ho VW, Leung K, Hsu A, et al.. A low-carbohydrate, high protein diet slows tumor growth and prevents cancer initiation. Cancer Research 2011 July;71(13);4484-93. <http://cancerres.aacrjournals.org/content/71/13/4484#F6>

may or may not be restricted in energy (caloric) content, depending on your appetite and goals (weight loss, weight maintenance, weight gain).

If you have a goal of weight loss, primal fasting can help you more easily achieve fat loss without loss of lean tissue. If you have a goal of weight maintenance, periodic fasting can help you maintain a lean condition without being obsessive about control of energy, fat, or even carbohydrate intake when you eat meals.

If you have a goal to gain some lean muscle tissue, primal fasting can help you prevent gaining fat as your weight increases.

An ancestrally-inspired, whole foods meat-based diet that includes regular periodic fasting may have the same or superior overall health and longevity benefits as chronic caloric restriction without the undesirable side effects of chronic energy deprivation.

3 The Mediterranean Diet: Feast or Fast?

By now, many people have heard that the Mediterranean diet confers health benefits. This idea came from studies of the people of Crete, done in the mid-20th century, which found that at that time, people living the traditional lifestyle of Crete had low rates of cardiovascular disease and cancer and greater longevity than any other nation known at the time.

Scientists and science writers in the media have attributed the relatively good health of the Cretan people to various foods found in their diet, such as olive oil, grapes and grape products (such as wine), whole grains, seafoods, walnuts, purslane, and others. People have been urged to consume more of these foods to improve their health.

The human mind tends to pay attention to and value the visible, and to not notice or value what is absent or invisible; and it tends to prefer adding to subtracting, gaining to losing. It considers "loser" an insult, even though sometimes losing is desirable, as in losing excess fat. Hence, we tend to focus on what the Mediterranean diet contains, not what it does not contain, and we like the idea of adding Mediterranean foods to our diet, more than the idea of subtracting foods from our diet.

This mental preference often makes us miss the mark. The benefits of the Cretan diet may lie largely in their not-eating practices, as opposed to their eating practices.

If you didn't know that fasting and food restrictions played an important role in the traditional, health-giving Mediterranean diet, I don't feel surprised. I have not seen a single popular report on the Mediterranean effect or diet that made any reference to fasting or caloric restriction.

Limited "fasting" resulting in significant caloric restriction played a very significant role in the traditional diet of Crete's people in times up to the mid-20th century when they were noted for their health and longevity.[19] A majority of people on Crete belonged to the Greek Orthodox Christian Church (GOC). This Church prescribes a total of 180–200 days of fasting – abstention from certain foods – per year.

Faithful Orthodox church members avoid olive oil, meat, fish, milk and dairy products every Wednesday and Friday (104 days) throughout the year. In addition, the Church specifies three principal fasting periods per year:

I. A total of 40 days preceding Christmas during which the faithful avoid eating meat, dairy products and eggs. During this time, the devout are allowed to eat fish and olive oil except on Wednesdays and Fridays.

II. A period of 48 days preceding Easter (Lent), during which fasters eat fish on only two days and olive oil only on weekends, and avoid meat, dairy products and eggs on all days.

---

[19] Sarri KO, Linardakis MK, Bervanaki FN, et al., "Greek Orthodox fasting rituals: a hidden characteristic of the Mediterranean diet of Crete," *Br J Nutr.* 2004 Aug;92(2):277-84. PubMed PMID: 15333159.

III.   A total of 15 days in August (the Assumption) having the same dietary rules as for Lent with the exception that one may consume fish only on August 6th.

Before you conclude that all these rules enforced a diet low in animal protein, you need to know that Orthodox fasting rituals allow unlimited high protein snails and seafood such as shrimps, squid, cuttlefish, octopus, lobsters, and crabs on all "fasting" days throughout the year.[20]

Note that on at least 104 days – more than one-quarter of days in the year – the faithful abstained from olive oil, the food that nevertheless has become the cardinal symbol of the Mediterranean diet.

Greek Orthodox fasting rituals produce energy restriction for the faithful on half of the days of the year. One study showed that people on Crete who followed the fasting rules of the GOC had, at the end of the food

---

[20] Sarri KO, Tzanakis NE, Linardakis MK, et al., "Effects of Greek orthodox christian church fasting on serum lipids and obesity," *BMC Public Health* 2003;3:16. <http://www.ncbi.nlm.nih.gov/pmc/articles/PMC156653/>

restriction periods, average caloric intakes of only about 1600 kcalories, almost 22% lower than Cretans who did not follow the "fasting" rules. Therefore, the original Mediterranean diet includes deliberate intermittent energy restriction, a fact rarely if ever mentioned by promoters of "the Mediterranean diet."

These people had an average caloric intake at least 30% lower than typical Americans eating 2400 or more calories daily. If they were healthier than typical Americans, was it because they ate the specific foods constituting "the Mediterranean diet," or because they mostly ate relatively nutrient-dense whole foods *and* less total food? Would a surplus-calorie "Mediterranean diet" produce the same health benefits? Probably not.

Although Greek Orthodox fasting does not necessarily involve prolonged periods on an absolute fast, it does result in limited food intake, which depletes stored glycogen and fat, reduces blood glucose and insulin levels, and allows cells and tissues to clear themselves of metabolic waste products. This chronic fasting/ energy restriction aspect of the traditional Cretan diet resonates with the intermittent energy restriction experienced by our ancestors. It may be the most powerful, yet overlooked aspect of the Mediterranean diet.

As discussed in later chapters, it appears that time-restricted feeding and periodic total fasting probably have benefits similar to chronic caloric restriction without restricting total energy intake.[21]

---

[21] Varady KA, Hellerstein MK. Alternate-day fasting and chronic disease prevention: a review of human and animal trials. Am J Clin Nutr 2007 July;86(1):7-13. <http://ajcn.nutrition.org/content/86/1/7.full>

4 Seventh Day Adventist Fasting

Seventh Day Adventists (SDAs) living in California have an average life expectancy about 9-10 years longer than non-SDA Californians.[22] Since vegan and vegetarian SDAs appear to live longer than non-vegetarian SDAs, advocates of plant-based diets have tended to exclusively credit abstention from animal foods for the reduced chronic disease risks and greater lifespan of SDAs.

It bears repeating that vegan and vegetarian diets are types of food restriction. A vegetarian avoids animal flesh; a vegan avoids all animal-source foods. SDAs who restrict foods of animal origin have a lower mean body mass index than those who do not. The greater the restriction of animal-source foods, the lower the body mass index, as shown in Table 4.1.[23]

---

[22] Fraser GE, Shavlik DJ, "Ten Years of Life: Is It a Matter of Choice?," *Arch Intern Med.* 2001;161(13):1645-1652. doi:10.1001/archinte.161.13.1645. <http://archinte.jamanetwork.com/article.aspx?articleid=648593>

[23] Rizzo NS, Jaceldo-Siegl K, Sabate J, Fraser GE. Nutrient Profiles of Vegetarian and Non Vegetarian Dietary Patterns. *Journal of the Academy of Nutrition and Dietetics.* 2013;113(12): 1610-1619. doi:10.1016/j.jand.2013.06.349. <https://www.ncbi.nlm.nih.gov/pmc/articles/PMC4081456/>

Table 4.1: Body mass index among Seventh Day Adventists according to vegetarian category.

Dietary category	Mean Body Mass Index
Non-vegetarian	28.6
Semi-vegetarian	27.4
Pesco-vegetarian	26.1
Lacto-ovo vegetarian	26.1
Vegan (strict vegetarian)	24.1

Thus, various levels of restriction of animal-source foods probably represent levels of dietary energy restriction. Since meat, eggs, and dairy products are nutrient- and energy-dense, vegetarians and vegans probably simply have a lower total energy intake than typical omnivores. Since dietary energy restriction appears to favor longevity in all animals, one must question whether the apparent reduced chronic disease risk and greater life span of SDAs is simply due to reduced total food energy intake, not specifically to avoidance of animal-source foods.

Advocates of plant-based diets believe that the vegetarian SDAs are healthier than non-vegetarians because they avoid "toxic" animal products, but the data is confounded by the fact that vegetarian SDAs apparently consume less total food energy and have lower mean body mass index. To support the idea that elimination of animal-source foods is the sole reason for the putative good health of SDAs, one would have to show that carnivores having lifestyles, mean total energy intakes and mean body mass indices comparable to vegan or vegetarian SDAs still have a higher disease risk and reduced life expectancy.[24] To my knowledge no one has ever shown this to be the case.

Most of the apparent greater longevity of Adventists is due to Adventist vegetarian men enjoying significantly reduced risk of cardiovascular disease mortality compared to non-vegetarian Adventists and non-Adventists. However, among Adventist women, total mortality rates are lowest among pesco-vegetarians and semi-vegetarians (who consumed non-fish meats

---

[24] Important lifestyle factors linked to reduced disease risk and greater longevity would include: non-smoking, low alcohol consumption, married with family, religious or other community support, physically active, adequate income, and positive social status, at a minimum.

1 time/mo or more and all animal flesh including fish at least 1 time/mo but no more than 1 time/wk).[25] This casts doubt on the idea that avoidance of animal foods is actually beneficial to Seventh Day Adventist women.

There is another factor in play. The SDA dietary guidelines include the suggestion to eat only two meals daily, which results in longer daily fasting periods than typical among non-SDA people.[26]

The founder of the SDA church, Ellen G. White, wrote:

"The stomach must have careful attention. It must not be kept in continual operation. Give this misused and much-abused organ some peace and quiet and rest. After the stomach has done its work for one meal, do not crowd more work upon it before it has had a chance to rest and before a sufficient supply

---

[25] Orlich MJ, Singh PN, Sabaté J, et al. Vegetarian Dietary Patterns and Mortality in Adventist Health Study 2. JAMA Intern Med 2013;173(13):1230-1238. <https://jamanetwork.com/journals/jamainternalmedicine/fullarticle/1710093> Data in Table 4.

[26] Kelly CJ, "A controlled trial of reduced meal frequency without caloric restriction in healthy, normal-weight, middle-aged adults," *Am J Clin Nutr* 2007 Oct; 86(4): 1254-1255. <http://ajcn.nutrition.org/content/86/4/1254.2.long>

of gastric juice is provided by nature to care for more food. Five hours at least should elapse between each meal, and always bear in mind that if you would give it a trial, you would find that two meals are better than three."[27]

White also recommended avoiding eating before sleeping and making breakfast – the first meal of the day, whenever it is taken – the most substantial meal.

"Another pernicious habit is that of eating just before bed-time. The regular meals may have been taken; but because there is a sense of faintness, more food is eaten. By indulgence, this wrong practice becomes a habit, and often so firmly fixed that it is thought impossible to sleep without food. As a result of eating late suppers, the digestive process is continued through the sleeping hours. But though the stomach works constantly, its work is not properly accomplished. The sleep is often disturbed with unpleasant dreams, and in the morning the person awakes unrefreshed, and with little relish for

---

[27] White EG. *Ellen G. White Writings*, Letter 73a, 1896. <https://text.egwwritings.org/publication.php?pubtype=Book&bookCode=CD&pagenumber=173>

breakfast. When we lie down to rest, the stomach should have its work all done, that it, as well as the other organs of the body, may enjoy rest. For persons of sedentary habits, late suppers are particularly harmful. With them the disturbance created is often the beginning of disease that ends in death."[28]

"It is the custom and order of society to take a slight breakfast. But this is not the best way to treat the stomach. At breakfast time the stomach is in a better condition to take care of more food than at the second or third meal of the day. The habit of eating a sparing breakfast and a large dinner is wrong. Make your breakfast correspond more nearly to the heartiest meal of the day."[29]

White's meal-timing advice – similar to that attributed to the legendary Siddhartha Gautama The Buddha –

---

[28] White EG. *Ellen G. White Writings*, The Ministry of Healing, 303-304. <https://text.egwwritings.org/publication.php?pubtype=Book&bookCode=TSDF&pagenumber=38>

[29] White EG. *Ellen G. White Writings* Letter 3, 1884. <https://text.egwwritings.org/publication.php?pubtype=Book&bookCode=CD&pagenumber=173>

has been supported by scientific research. Some research indicates that animals and people who consume most of their food late in their normal waking period have greater body fat and more metabolic disorders than those who consume most of their food early in the normal waking period (i.e. early in daylight hours for humans).[30, 31]

People assigned to consume most of their calories early in the day (700 kcal breakfast, 500 kcal lunch, 200 kcal supper) showed less hunger, greater satiety, and greater reductions of body weight, waist circumference, serum triglycerides, fasting glucose, fasting insulin, and insulin resistance than those assigned to eat most of their food late in the day (200

---

[30] Ibid.

[31] Fuse Y, Hirao A, Kuroda H, et al., "Differential roles of breakfast only (one meal per day) and a bigger breakfast with a small dinner (two meals per day) in mice fed a high-fat diet with regard to induced obesity and lipid metabolism," *Journal of Circadian Rhythms*, 10, p.Art. 4. DOI: http://doi.org/10.1186/1740-3391-10-4 <http://www.jcircadianrhythms.com/articles/10.1186/1740-3391-10-4/>

kcal breakfast, 500 kcal lunch, 700 kcal dinner) for 12 weeks.[32] I discuss this further in chapter 9.

Typically, SDAs who implement the two-meal plan eat breakfast and lunch. This pattern is also recommended by Chinese medicine, which acknowledges greater digestive efficiency in the morning and noon hours, but greater storage efficiency in the evening hours. In fact some chronobiology research resonates with the Chinese medical view, indicating that the stomach is significantly more active at 8 a.m. than 8 p.m., taking 50% more time to empty in the evening than in the morning.[33] The authors of this study suggested that people who have problems with indigestion and acid reflux disease should eat less food in the evening.

Assuming these two meals occur within about 4 to 8 hours of each other, this would result in daily fasting periods of 16 to 20 hours. This time-restricted feeding

---

[32] Jakubowicz D, Barnea M, et al., "High Caloric intake at breakfast vs. dinner differentially influences weight loss of overweight and obese women," *Obesity* 2013 Dec;21(12);2504-2512. <http://onlinelibrary.wiley.com/doi/10.1002/oby.20460/full>

[33] Goo RH, Moore JG, Greenberg E, Alazraki NP. Circadian Variation in Gastric Emptying of Meals in Humans. Gastroenterology 1987 Sep;93(3):513-8.

(TRF) regimen very likely results in an lower total food energy intake and other metabolic benefits (discussed in chapter 7) for SDA vegetarians and confounds the association between reduced animal food consumption and lower disease risk among SDAs.

Do SDA vegetarians have better health because they avoid animal foods, because they eat less food energy (calories) overall, or because they spend more time in a fasted state and less time in the fed state? I have never seen any research addressing this question. However, a comparison with members of the Church of Latter Day Saints, or Mormons, may shed some light on this question. Mormons have similar lifestyles to SDAs, but they do not avoid meat, and they do practice periodic fasting, typically a 24-hour fast once monthly, and they start this habit in children as young as 8 years of age. Research has demonstrated that meat-eating Mormons who regularly practice this fasting ritual have a significantly reduced risk of atherosclerotic heart disease and diabetes compared to Mormons who have similar lifestyles and diets but don't adhere to the fasting ritual.[34] This suggests that even very limited absolute fasting has a very profound beneficial effect on health. Hence, the habitual time-restricted feeding regimen of many SDA vegetarians and vegans could account for the lower cardiovascular disease and other mortality rates among SDA men.

Why might vegetarian SDA women fare poorly compared to men and those SDA women who eat animal products? Women have higher dietary requirements for iron and other nutrients due to menstruation, pregnancy and lactation, so they are more prone to disease due to deficiencies when eating a diet restricted in either total energy (kcalories) or animal foods – the best sources of blood-building nutrients. Animal studies indicate that combining dietary energy restriction with intermittent fasting will disrupt hormonal cycles in females.[35] Vegetarian SDA

---

[34] Horne BD, May HT, Anderson JL, et al., "Usefulness of Routine Periodic Fasting to Lower Risk of Coronary Artery Disease among Patients Undergoing Coronary Angiography," *Am J Cardiology* 2008;102(7):814-819. doi:10.1016/j.amjcard.2008.05.021. <www.ncbi.nlm.nih.gov/pmc/articles/PMC2572991/>

[35] Kumar S, Kaur G. Intermittent Fasting Dietary Restriction Regimen Negatively Influences Reproduction in Young Rats: A Study of Hypothalamo-Hypophysial-Gonadal Axis. PLOS One 2013 Jan 29 <https://doi.org/10.1371/journal.pone.0052416>

women have a five times greater risk of menstrual irregularity (i.e. hormonal deficiency) than non-vegetarians; dietary animal protein and cholesterol protect women from this disruption.[36] Women should not combine fasting or time-restricted feeding with restriction of energy or meat and egg intake.

[36] Pedersen AB, Bartholomew MJ, Dolence LA, et al.. Menstrual differences due to vegetarian and nonvegetarian diets. Am J Clin Nutr 1991;53:879-85.

5 Feeding & Fasting: Yin & Yang

In the universal theory of Chinese science, the terms yin and yang[37] simply represent two types of phenomena presented in our experience. Applied as a medical theory, every physiological disorder results from an imbalance between yin and yang influences.

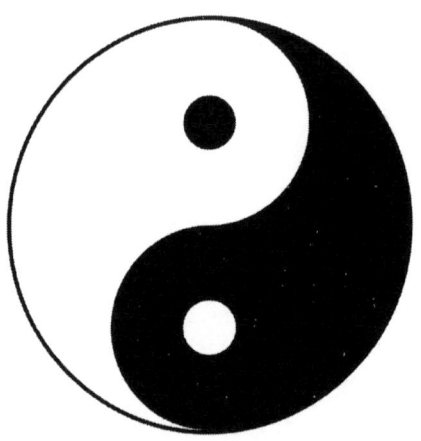

Simply put, phenomena which we experience as relatively cool, quiet, slow, dark, soft and moist belong to the yin category, and those which we experience as relatively warm, loud, fast, bright, hard and dry belong to the yang category. The classic *tàijí* (太極; literally: "great pole") symbol – more commonly known as the

---

[37] Properly pronounced "yeen" and "yahng."

yin-yang symbol – represents graphically the annual, seasonal variation in Solar energy reaching the Earth,[38] so depicts the bipolarity of phenomena. In this symbol, yang is represented by the white domains (representing the increase of light and energy that occurs over the spring and summer), and yin by the black domains (representing the waning of light and energy that occurs over the fall and winter). The fact that each phase contains the seed of its opposite is depicted by the opposite-colored dots within the waxing (largest) portion of each phase.

When the body has too much exposure to yin influences and not enough to yang influences, it becomes too yin itself; and vice versa, when it has too much exposure to yang influences and not enough to yin, it becomes too yang. Food is moist and material, so feeding produces a more yin condition, whereas fasting and exercise burn up food and discharge fluids

---

[38] The graph is obtained obtained by plotting on a compass the lengths and positions of the shadows cast at noon, day after day for an entire year, by a pole posted at right angles to ground. Jaeger S. A Geomedical Approach to Chinese Medicine: The Origin of the Yin-Yang Symbol. In: Recent Advances in Theories and Practice of Chinese Medicine, ed. By Haixue Kuang. Intech, 2012

(through sweating) so they produce a more yang condition.

This is confirmed by Western physiology, which reports that in the fed state the body shifts into a rest-and-digest mode of accumulating matter and energy that is ruled by the parasympathetic nervous system.

Eating carbohydrates stimulates the pancreas to release the hormone insulin, which drives sugar, amino acids, and fatty acids out of the blood into cells, and stimulates the build-up (expansion) of glycogen, protein, and fat stores. Insulin also causes the kidneys to retain both sodium and water, leading to water retention. After carbohydrate-rich meals the body tends to feel bloated, heavy and lethargic, the mind is more dull, and there is a natural tendency to sleepiness.

In the normal fasted state the sympathetic nervous system becomes dominant and the body converts stored matter to energy. During a fast the pancreas releases the hormone glucagon, which has opposite effects of insulin, stimulating the breakdown of fats and glycogen. As insulin levels drop, fatty acids are released from adipose and glycogen from liver and muscle, and these are metabolized for energy. When insulin drops low enough, the kidneys release sodium and water follows.

Consequently, the body feels lighter and energetic, the mind is more alert, and there is a natural tendency to physical and mental activity. In the fasted state, matter (in the forms of glycogen and fatty acids) is converted into energy and dispersed outward. As body water, glycogen and fat stores contract, the body becomes leaner, denser, and harder. Hence, short-term fasting makes the body and mind more yang: light and energetic; while overeating makes one more yin: dull and lethargic.

On the other hand, excessive food restriction will create nutritional deficiencies. To maintain health, one must balance yin and yang Influences, intake and expenditure. Neither overeating nor excessive food restriction is beneficial in the long run. Primal fasting allows you to easily strike a healthy balance between excess and deficiency.

6 Physiology of Fasting

After a meal, your body shifts into a period of digestion and absorption that lasts for about 3 hours; in this fed state, the body uses the carbohydrates, fat, and proteins from the food to replenish energy stores depleted during fasting or exercise. If glycogen stores have been depleted (by fasting or exercise), carbohydrates will first get stored as glycogen, both in the liver and in the muscles, but if glycogen stores are full, the extra carbohydrate (starch or sugar) will get converted to fat.

From roughly 3 to about 12-18 hours after a meal, your body operates in the post-absorptive or early fasting state. In the early part of this stage, the body cells derive much of their energy needs from breakdown of stored carbohydrate (glycogen – the bulk of which was supplied by the last meal) and/or body fat.

Depending on the size of your last meal, sometime in the period between 12 and 18 hours after that meal you transition to fasting metabolism, which continues up to about 48 hours. During this stage, between about

15 and 48 hours past the last meal, your body shifts to getting an increasing proportion of its energy from fat — one of the main goals of the anyone seeking fat loss.

Metabolic changes that produce other major health benefits of fasting also occur in this stage. During this phase you get these beneficial changes (discussed in the next chapter), without incurring major losses of lean healthy tissue (such as muscle), or metabolic power, so long as you get food by the end of 48 hours.

If you go without eating for more than about 72 hours, your metabolism shifts to the long-term fasting or starvation stage. At this stage, you may start to see losses in lean tissue. I recommend that you generally avoid fasting more than 36 hours, so you get all the benefits of fasting, but never incur the losses involved in starving.

7 Beneficial Metabolic Effects of Fasting

Regular moderate-length periods of fasting (15-24 hours) can help you achieve the lean and healthy body you desire, because it has numerous beneficial metabolic effects.

1. Glycogen depletion

Humans have no dietary requirement for carbohydrate[39] because the liver can convert a part of the fats and a part of the protein we eat into blood sugar on demand. It seems likely that Nature granted us this ability precisely because our habitual ancestral diet had little or no carbohydrate for extended periods

---

[39] Food and Nutrition Board, National Academy of Sciences. Dietary Reference Intakes for Energy, Carbohydrate, Fiber, Fat, Fatty Acids, Cholesterol, Protein, and Amino Acids. National Academies Press, 2005. Pages 275-6. "The lower limit of dietary carbohydrate compatible with life apparently is zero, provided that adequate amounts of protein and fat are consumed." <https://www.nap.edu/read/10490/chapter/8?term=carbohydrate+requirement#275>

of time during the Ice Ages when our ancestors subsisted primarily on animal protein and fat.[40, 41, 42]

When dietary carbohydrate is minimal or absent, the liver has total control of the blood sugar level, and keeps it very stable. At any point in time, the human blood stream contains only about 5 grams – that's about 1 teaspoon – of sugar.

A medium fruit contains about 25 grams (5 teaspoons) of sugar, one slice of homemade whole grain bread

---

40 Richards MP. A brief review of the archaeological evidence for Palaeolithic and Neolithic subsistence. Eur J Clin Nutr. 2002 Dec; 56(12):16 p following 1262. PubMed PMID: 12494313.

[41] Senckenberg Research Institute and Natural History Museum. "Neanderthals diet: 80% meat, 20% vegetables: Isotope studies shed a new light on the eating habits of the prehistoric humans." ScienceDaily. ScienceDaily, 14 March 2016. <www.sciencedaily.com/releases/2016/03/160314091128.htm>. Citation: Christoph Wißing, Hélène Rougier, Isabelle Crevecoeur, Mietje Germonpré, Yuichi I. Naito, Patrick Semal, Hervé Bocherens. Isotopic evidence for dictary ecology of late Neandertals in North-Western Europe. Quaternary International, 2015; DOI: 10.1016/j.quaint.2015.09.091

[42] Ben-Dor M, Gopher A, Hershkovitz I, Barkai R. Man the Fat Hunter: The Demise of Homo erectus and the Emergence of a New Hominin Lineage in the Middle Pleistocene (ca. 400 kyr) Levant. Smith FH, ed. PLoS ONE. 2011;6(12):e28689. doi: 10.1371/journal.pone.0028689. <https://www.ncbi.nlm.nih.gov/pmc/articles/PMC3235142/>

contains about 10 grams (2 teaspoons), a large potato about 54 grams (10 teaspoons!) and a half cup of rice (brown or white) contains about 20 grams (4 teaspoons). A single-serving of high carbohydrate food can result in a dramatic increase in blood sugar levels, by-passing the liver's careful regulation of the blood sugar level.

To prevent metabolic emergency from sudden surges in blood sugar due to carbohydrate consumption, the liver and muscles convert the excess dietary carbohydrate into a type of starch called glycogen. The liver can store about 100 g of glycogen, and the muscles 300 to 400 g.

When your glycogen stores are full, your cells increase their use of carbohydrate and reduce their use of fat for fuel. This means that you must deplete your glycogen stores in order to to activate maximum fat burning.

How can you deplete glycogen? We have three very effective ways:

1. **Limit your dietary carbohydrate to less than 75** g **per day.** This reduces both muscle and liver glycogen.
2. Engage in brief bouts of very high intensity exercise, such as resistance training or sprinting, alternating 20-90 second periods of heavy exertion with 60-180 second periods of rest for about 10-20 minutes. This depletes muscle glycogen.
3. **Fast (water-only) for at least 16 hours.** This primarily depletes liver glycogen. However, if you do this daily and combine with a reduced carbohydrate intake and high intensity exercise, you will also gradually reduce habitual muscle glycogen levels and maintain them at a reduced level, keeping your system in a fat-burning mode.

Since 16 hours of fasting significantly depletes liver glycogen stores, implementing daily fasts of 14-16 hours will improve your ability to utilize body fat as fuel, and can help you reduce your daily total food energy intake to reduce body fat stores.

Alternatively, you can implement a couple of 24 hour fasts each week to achieve the same goals, or combine the two approaches to fit your lifestyle. I fast 14-16 hours every day, and fast 24 hours or more whenever my appetite dictates, usually about 1-3 times a month.

If you exercise intensely during the last couple of hours of a fast lasting at least 16 hours, your ratio of energy output to energy intake is maximized at the same time that glycogen is maximally depleted.

2. Increased insulin sensitivity

Research has demonstrated that a 16 hour fast improves insulin sensitivity of muscle cells, which means that when you do eat carbohydrates, they will get channeled more effectively to your muscle cells for use as fuel or to be stored as glycogen, rather than getting channeled to fat cells to get converted to fat.[43] Improving insulin sensitivity is a key goal in preventing and treating type 2 diabetes (NIDDM).

---

[43] Heijboer AC, Donga E, Voshol PJ, et al., "Sixteen hours of fasting differentially affects hepatic and muscle insulin sensitivity in mice," *J Lipid Res* 2005;46:582-588.

By the end of a 24 hour fast, blood insulin levels drop by about 35%, and over 72 hours, they drop by more than 50%.[44] You want this to happen because insulin stimulates fat storage and blocks fat burning, so reduced insulin levels translates to reduced fat storage and increased fat burning.

Regular fasting also improves insulin sensitivity. After a 15 day period during which subjects fasted 20 hours every alternate day, but ate abundantly on other days and did not lose body fat (i.e. no net energy restriction), insulin sensitivity improved markedly.[45] Insulin insensitivity plays a role in diabetes type 2, so intermittent fasting can help prevent or reverse this disease. Increased insulin sensitivity results in lower insulin production, hence better fat metabolism.

---

[44] Klein S, et al., "Progressive Alterations in lipid and glucose metabolism durlng short-term fasting in young adult men," *Am J Physiology* 1993; 265 (Endocrinology and metabolism 28):E801-E806 <http://ajpendo.physiology.org/content/ajpendo/265/5/E801.full.pdf>

[45] Halberg N, Henriksen M, Söderhamn N, et al., "Effect of intermittent fasting and refeeding on insulin action in healthy men," *J Appl Physiol* 99:2128-2136, 2005. <http://jap.physiology.org/content/99/6/2128.long>

3. Increases in fat-metabolizing enzymes

As you enter a fasted, glycogen-depleted state, your body cells rapidly increase their production of enzymes involved in burning fat. The body fat cells release fat into the blood stream, and the muscle cells—the primary fat burners in the body—start sucking the fat out of the blood stream to burn for fuel.

The muscle cells use an enzyme called uncoupling protein-3 (UCP3) when burning fat. Fifteen hours of fasting raises the level of UCP3 five-fold, and by 40 hours the level has increased by more than 10-fold![46]

At the end of 24 hours of fasting, release of fat from fat cells and use of fat by muscle cells increases by 50%, and most of this increase occurs between 18 and 24 hours. When you fast regularly (once or twice weekly) the body adapts by keeping levels of fat burning

---

[46] Tunstall RJ, et al., "Fasting activates the gene expression of UCP3 independent of genes necessary for lipid transport and oxidation in skeletal muscle," *Biochem Biophys Res Comm* 2002; 294:301-308

enzymes elevated at all times. Periodic fasting literally turns your body into a fat-burning machine.

4. Lipolysis

About 12 to 18 hours into a period of water-only fasting, lipolysis, the breakdown of fat, becomes the major energy pathway. As blood sugar reaches normal fasting levels, the body responds by releasing glucagon and epinephrine (adrenaline), and these hormones act to stimulate the breakdown of fat and increase the cells' use of fat as fuel. The increased levels of epinephrine also give you a sense of mental clarity and energy not available in the fed state without taking drugs like caffeine.

As the cells metabolize fats in a carbohydrate-restricted condition, they convert the fats to ketones, a process called ketosis. Whereas glucose (from starch, sugar, or glycogen) has only 4 calories per gram, ketones supply 4.6 calories per gram. In an individual not adapted to fasting, all tissues of the body except for red blood cells and the central nervous tissue can use ketones for fuel. (The brain can adapt to using ketones after prolonged fasting.[47]) During the period between 16 and 36 hours of a fast the body reserves any available glucose for the red blood cells and central nervous system, and adapts to burning ketones in other tissues, so you won't lack energy during brief absolute fasts.

If you exercise during a fast, your muscle cells will burn fat for fuel at a higher rate than if you exercise in a fed state.

Since fat burning increases dramatically during a fast, even without changing the types of foods you eat on non-fasting days, fasting facilitates rapid fat loss. The average largely sedentary person expends 1500 to 2500 calories daily in life maintenance and activities, and one pound of stored fat contains 3500 calories. If the average largely sedentary individual abstains from food for a whole day each week, and eats normally on non-fasting days, he or she can lose one-half to two-thirds of a pound of fat each week; and if this individual

[47] Owen OE, "Ketone bodies as a fuel for the brain during starvation," *Biochem Mol Biol Educ* 2005 Jul;33(4):246-51. <http://onlinelibrary.wiley.com/doi/10.1002/bmb.2005.49403304246/full>

fasted two days of each week, he or she could lose at least one pound of fat in the week.

Remember, you can achieve those results just by fasting. If you eat a low carbohydrate whole foods meat-based diet, you may lose fat even more rapidly.

5. Brown fat activation

Humans have two types of fat: white, which has little metabolic activity, and brown (or beige) which actively burns fat to generate heat (thermogenesis). Intermittent fasting reshapes the gut microbiome (flora) in a way that induces beiging of white fat, which increases thermogenesis and reverses metabolic disorder.[48]

6. Increased human growth hormone (hGH) release

One of the most remarkable effects of fasting consists of dramatic increases in the release of human growth

---

[48] LI G, Xie C, Lu S, et al. Intermittent Fasting Promotes White Adipose Browning and Decreases Obesity by Shaping the Gut Microbiota. Cell Metab 2017 Oct 3;26(4):672-85.e4.

hormone.[49, 50] People presently spend thousands of dollars monthly for injections of growth hormone to reverse the effects of aging, but they could get increased exposure to growth hormone without monetary expense by simply fasting once or twice weekly, or 16-23 hours daily.

The pituitary gland releases GH in pulses throughout the day. Fasting for just 24 hours has a dramatic effect on GH output; it increases the frequency of GH pulses by 25%, it doubles the peak amplitude of GH pulses, and it quadruples the interpeak serum GH levels.[51]

Growth hormone stimulates breakdown of fat, growth of muscle, and repair of tissues and DNA. For this reason, regular fasting or time-restricted feeding may

---

[49] Ho KY, Veldhuis JD, Johnson ML, et al., "Fasting enhances growth hormone secretion and amplifies the complex rhythms of growth hormone secretion in man," *Journal of Clinical Investigation* 1988;81(4):968-975. <http://www.ncbi.nlm.nih.gov/pmc/articles/PMC329619/>

[50] Kerndt PR, Naughton JL, Driscoll CE, Loxterkamp DA, "Fasting: The History, Pathophysiology and Complications." *Western Journal of Medicine* 1982;137(5):379-399. <http://www.ncbi.nlm.nih.gov/pmc/articles/PMC1274154/>

[51] Ho KY, et al.. Op. cit..

make you look and feel younger, lose fat, and build muscle.

An 8 week long human study compared the effects of eating all caloric requirements in just one as opposed to the conventional three meals per day.[52] This study found that the people assigned to fasting 20 hours daily, then eating all of their caloric requirements in only 1 evening meal each day lost an average of 1.4 kg (3 lb.) body mass and 2.1 kg (4.6 lb.) fat mass over the eight weeks, which means that they gained an average of 1.6 lb. lean mass over the study period, with no change in exercise habits. If not experimental error, this increase in lean mass may have resulted from increased GH output during the long fasting periods daily. The results of this study were supported in a study which found that mice subjected to energy and macronutrient restriction had higher bone density and

---

[52] Stote KS, Baer DJ, Spears K, et al., "A controlled trial of reduced meal frequency without caloric restriction in healthy, normal-weight, middle-aged adults," *The Am J Clin Nutr* 2007;85(4):981-988. <http://www.ncbi.nlm.nih.gov/pmc/articles/PMC2645638/>

no age-related loss of muscle mass compared to mice fed ad libitum.[53]

7. Elimination of excess sodium and water

Elevated insulin levels cause your body to retain sodium and water. Fasting (and low carbohydrate intake) lowers your insulin level, and this causes natriuresis, the elimination of sodium, and water, through urination. This relieves edema and eliminates that puffy, doughy appearance you don't like.

8. Reduced oxidative stress and inflammation

One of the most important ketones has the name ß-hydroxybutyrate (BHB). As noted, as a ketone, BHB releases more energy per gram than glucose. In addition, BHB counteracts neurotoxins capable of causing Parkinson's and Alzheimer's diseases and

---

[53] Van Norren K, Rusli F, van Dijk M, et al., "Behavioural changes are a major contributing factor in the reduction of sarcopenia in caloric-restricted ageing mice," *Journal of Cachexia, Sarcopenia and Muscle* 2015;6(3):253-268. doi:10.1002/jcsm.12024.

counters free radical damage.[54, 55] BHB also has a strong anti-inflammatory effect.[56]

Overweight asthma patients who adhered to 8 weeks of alternate day 80% caloric restriction experienced significant sustained decreases in serum levels of several markers of oxidative stress and inflammation,[57] including C-reactive protein (C-RP), interleukin-6 (IL-6), tumor necrosis factor-alpha, ceramides, leptin, and serum brain-derived neurotrophic factor (BDNF).

---

[54] Tieu K, Perier C, Caspersen C, et al., "D-β-Hydroxybutyrate rescues mitochondrial respiration and mitigates features of Parkinson disease," *J Clin Invest* 2003;112(6):892-901. doi: 10.1172/JCI200318797. <http://www.ncbi.nlm.nih.gov/pmc/articles/PMC193668/>

[55] Kashiwaya Y, Takeshima T, Mori N, et al., "d-β-Hydroxybutyrate protects neurons in models of Alzheimer's and Parkinson's disease," *Proceedings of the National Academy of Sciences of the United States of America* 2000;97(10):5440-5444. <http://www.ncbi.nlm.nih.gov/pmc/articles/PMC25847/>

[56] Youm Y-H, Nguyen KY, Grant RW, et al. Ketone body β-hydroxybutyrate blocks the NLRP3 inflammasome-mediated inflammatory disease. *Nature medicine.* 2015;21(3):263-269. doi: 10.1038/nm.3804. <https://www.ncbi.nlm.nih.gov/pmc/articles/PMC4352123/>

[57] Johnson J et al, "Alternate day calorie restriction improves clinical findings and reduces markers of oxidative stress and inflammation in overweight adults with moderate asthma," *Free Radic Biol Med* 2007 Mar 1;42(5):665-74. Epub 2006 Dec 14. <http://www.ncbi.nlm.nih.gov/pmc/articles/PMC1859864/>

Serum levels of TNF alpha declined by about 60%, BDNF by about 70%.

In this same study, markers of oxidative stress also declined dramatically. For example, levels of protein carbonyls and 8-isoprostane fell 80%, nitrotyrosine fell more than 90%, and 4-hydroxynonenal adducts fell about 50%.

In addition, studies show that global cell proliferation declines on 24/24 fast/feast programs. This means fasting 24 hours stops the growth of rogue cells that could become tumors, cysts, or cancers, and reduces cell proliferation characteristic of atherosclerosis and some other diseases like psoriasis.

9. Healing of gut inflammation and leakage

Diets rich in ground grains, refined carbohydrates or vegetable oils increase the risk of inflammation of the gut, whereas diets rich in whole animal foods (meat, eggs, milk) reduce gut inflammation.[58, 59] As this progresses, the gut becomes leaky, allowing incompletely digested nutrients to enter the blood stream. Once these incompletely digested nutrients enter the blood, the white blood cells mount an attack on them, causing inflammation and making you feel sick. Some of the cells make antibodies to the foreign proteins, and if these proteins have sufficient similarity to proteins in your own tissues, the antibodies will proceed to attack your own tissues, causing autoimmune diseases.

---

[58] Spreadbury I. Comparison with ancestral diets suggests dense acellular carbohydrates promote an inflammatory microbiota, and may be the primary dietary cause of leptin resistance and obesity. *Diabetes, Metabolic Syndrome and Obesity: Targets and Therapy.* 2012;5:175-189. doi:10.2147/DMSO.S33473. <https://www.ncbi.nlm.nih.gov/pmc/articles/PMC3402009/>

[59] Youm Y-H, Nguyen KY, Grant RW, et al. Ketone body β-hydroxybutyrate blocks the NLRP3 inflammasome-mediated inflammatory disease. *Nature medicine.* 2015;21(3):263-269. doi:10.1038/nm.3804. <https://www.ncbi.nlm.nih.gov/pmc/articles/PMC4352123/>

Fasting may decrease intestinal permeability (leakage) and thus be beneficial for disorders involving leaky gut such as autoimmune diseases.[60]

10. Central nervous system (CNS) improvements

Fasting improves a number of aspects of brain health and function.[61, 62] It protects brain neurons from stressors, including chemical toxins. While fasting decreases the amount of brain-derived neurotrophic factor in the blood – a good sign – it increases the amount of brain-derived neurotrophic factor where it belongs, in the brain itself, which promotes healthy

---

[60] Sunqvist T, Lindstrom F, Magnusson KE, et al., "Influence of fasting on intestinal permeability and disease activity in patients with rheumatoid arthritis," *Scand J Rheumatol* 1082;11(1):33-8. Abstract.

[61] Longo VD, Mattson MP, "Fasting: Molecular Mechanisms and Clinical Applications," *Cell metabolism* 2014;19(2):181-192. doi: 10.1016/j.cmet.2013.12.008. <http://www.ncbi.nlm.nih.gov/pmc/articles/PMC3946160/>

[62] Mattson MP, Duan W, Guo Z, "Meal size and frequency affect neuronal plasticity and vulnerability to disease: cellular and molecular mechanisms, *J Neurochem* 2003;84:417-31. <http://onlinelibrary.wiley.com/doi/10.1046/j.1471-4159.2003.01586.x/epdf>

growth of brain neurons and has an antidepressant effect. Fasting after a brain injury improves neuronal recovery. There exists evidence that dietary restriction reduces the negative effects of vitamin or mineral deficiency on the nervous system.[63] Numerous animal studies show that fasting improves learning and delays brain aging. Thus, it is likely that regular periodic fasting will help protect you from neurodegenerative diseases like Alzheimer's dementia and Parkinson's disease. As already noted, adherence to a low carbohydrate diet may have similar effects, because limiting dietary carbohydrate induces a metabolic state similar to fasting (low blood glucose and insulin,

---

[63] Ibid.

increased cellular levels of ketones, including BHB).[64,] [65, 66]

11. Sensory enhancement

Fasting causes a rapid change in the sensitivity of sensory organs. Frequent feeding dulls the sense organs, especially if one's habitual food has high sugar contents or intense flavoring with salt or spices. After a fast, your sense of taste and appreciation of subtle flavors dramatically improves. This helps you to break an addiction to high fat, high sugar, highly seasoned

---

[64] Manninen AH. Metabolic Effects of the Very-Low-Carbohydrate Diets: Misunderstood "Villains" of Human Metabolism. *Journal of the International Society of Sports Nutrition*. 2004;1(2):7-11. doi: 10.1186/1550-2783-1-2-7. <https://www.ncbi.nlm.nih.gov/pmc/articles/PMC2129159/>

[65] Youm Y-H, Nguyen KY, Grant RW, et al. Ketone body β-hydroxybutyrate blocks the NLRP3 inflammasome-mediated inflammatory disease. *Nature medicine*. 2015;21(3):263-269. doi: 10.1038/nm.3804. <https://www.ncbi.nlm.nih.gov/pmc/articles/PMC4352123/>

[66] Cotter DG, Schugar RC, Crawford PA. Ketone body metabolism and cardiovascular disease. *American Journal of Physiology - Heart and Circulatory Physiology*. 2013;304(8):H1060-H1076. doi: 10.1152/ajpheart.00646.2012. <https://www.ncbi.nlm.nih.gov/pmc/articles/PMC3625904/>

processed foods so that you can adopt a higher quality whole foods diet.

12. Cellular Cleansing

The normal process of metabolism of nutrients produces free radicals, which damage proteins and organelles in our cells, resulting in the effects we associate with aging. This damage particularly affects the mitochondria, the energy-generating organelles in every cell. If the cells don't remove damaged, malfunctioning mitochondria, the latter begin to spew out suicidal proteins prompting the entire cell to die. The aging process consists of this death of cells.

When fasted for 16 or more hours, your cells switch to a self-cleansing mode called *autophagy* where they release enzymes that digest the metabolic waste accumulated during the fed state, such as damaged proteins and injured mitochondria, and recycle their building blocks into new cellular materials.[67]

---

[67] Mattson MP, Allison DB, Fontana L, et al., "Meal frequency and timing in health and disease," *Proceedings of the National Academy of Sciences of the United States of America* 2014;111(47):16647-16653. doi:10.1073/pnas.1413965111.

Fasting also allows your fat cells to release the fat-soluble toxins they store. These then travel to the liver, which detoxifies the stuff and sends it out of the body through bile.

13. Possible increased lifespan

If you fast regularly, but not too often, you may live longer than if you do not fast. In humans, periodic fasting or caloric restriction activates the SIRT1 gene.[68] SIRT1 acts as a "rescue gene" that initiates repair of free radical damage, prevents premature cell death, increases energy production by mitochondria (cellular power generators), inhibits fat storage, stimulates fat catabolism, and reduces inflammation and oxidative stress.

Animal studies have demonstrated that periodically fasted animals live longer than their non-fasted peers. For example, in 1945, Anton Carlson and Frederick Hoelzel, both from the University of Chicago Department of Physiology, published a report of their

---

[68] Mattson MP, Duan W, Guo Z, op. cit..

experiments with intermittent fasting of rats.[69] They tested the effects of fasting 1 day in 2, 1 day in 3, and 1 day in 4; the rats ate freely, without any restrictions, on non-fast days. The results indicated that for the average rat the 1 day in 3 provided the optimum amount of fasting; 1 day in 2 and 1 day in 4 led to early demise for many rats. Among rats fasted 1 day in 3, the average male rat's lifespan increased by 20%, and the average female's by 15%, compared to non-fasted rats. That would translate to a 12 to 20 year gain in lifespan for a human.

In a 1957 Spanish study of elders, those who engaged in alternate day semi-fasting (~50% caloric restriction days alternated with ~50% caloric surplus days) were half as likely to die over a three-year period. Also, those who fasted spent only 123 days in a hospital,

---

[69] Carlson AJ, Hoelzel F, "Apparent prolongation of the life span of rats by intermittent fasting," *J Nutr* 1946 March 1;31(3):363-375. <http://jn.nutrition.org/content/31/3/363.extract>

compared to 219 days for those who ate as much as they wanted every day.[70]

As already mentioned, Mormons who fast once a month have a significantly reduced risk of atherosclerotic heart disease and diabetes – two of the leading causes of premature death in modern nations – compared to Mormons who have similar lifestyles and diets but don't adhere to the fasting ritual.[71] Finally, SDAs, many of whom practice time-restricted feeding, have an average life expectancy about 9-10 years longer than non-SDA Californians.[72]

---

[70] Johnson JB, Laub DR, John S, "The effect on health of alternate day calorie restriction: Eating less and more than needed on alternate days prolongs life," *Medical Hypotheses* 2006;67:209-211. <http://www.johnsonupdaydowndaydiet.com/pdf/ADCR%20JBJ%20MH.pdf>

[71] Horne BD, May HT, Anderson JL, et al., "Usefulness of Routine Periodic Fasting to Lower Risk of Coronary Artery Disease among Patients Undergoing Coronary Angiography," *Am J Cardiology* 2008;102(7):814-819. doi:10.1016/j.amjcard.2008.05.021. <www.ncbi.nlm.nih.gov/pmc/articles/PMC2572991/>

[72] Fraser GE, Shavlik DJ, "Ten Years of Life: Is It a Matter of Choice?," *Arch Intern Med.* 2001;161(13):1645-1652. doi:10.1001/archinte.161.13.1645. <http://archinte.jamanetwork.com/article.aspx?articleid=648593>

Thus, time-restricted feeding and periodic 24 hour fasting, even just once a month, probably increase your chances for realizing a longer healthy lifespan.

8 Fasting & Human Performance

Many people believe that one should eat something before engaging in mental or physical activity in order to ensure that you have sufficient energy to complete the task. The idea is that the energy you need for high performance comes from your most recent meal.

This is a myth. A pretty large meal will provide about 1000 kcal. In comparison, after an overnight fasting period of 16-18 hours, the average lean person can have some 1500 to 2000 kcal stored as glycogen (carbohydrate), and at least 37,000 kcal of total energy reserves (glycogen and fat). A meal or snack is a drop in the bucket of your total body energy stores. Further, food intake primarily goes to replenish depleted energy (glycogen and fat) stores, not directly to use for ongoing energy needs.

You will not "run out of energy" for physical or mental activity just 16, 20, 24, 36, or even 48 hours after eating. You would have to go without food for 90 days or more to totally deplete your body's energy reserves.

All wild animals, including our hunting and gathering ancestors, had to perform demanding mental and physical tasks in order to acquire fresh food after fasting overnight. If ancient humans had been unable to hunt and gather when hungry, they would have perished and we would not exist today. In natural habitats, natural selection favors the survival and reproduction of individuals who can function at a high level in the food quest when hungry. We are descended from those ancient humans who excelled at food acquisition even if they had to go a few days without eating. Those ancient humans who could not function well on an empty stomach were unsuccessful hunters and foragers when times got lean, and therefore they perished or left few descendants compared to those who could bring home some bison even if they hadn't had a meal in a few days.

I once believed that I would be unable to do heavy physical training on an empty stomach, and would make sure that I scheduled my heavy training sessions after meals. However, after experimenting with training in a fasted state, I realized that eating before training had never given me significant benefit.

In fact, if eating before training had any effect on my performance at all, it was likely to be negative, in the form of stomach cramps or discomfort while working hard, particularly if sprinting, falling and rolling (martial arts), or doing movements that require strong abdominal muscle activation. I have found that I function best in physical training if I do it toward the end of my 16-20 hour overnight fast (which currently is usually in the morning).

Kohei Uchimura, perhaps the greatest male gymnast of all-time – a two-time Olympic all-around champion and six-time world all around winner – eats only one meal a day, in the evening, after his two workouts.[73] He came upon this regimen because he doesn't like to have a full stomach when he is training. He explained:

> "In gymnastics, you spin around a lot, right?
> So I get sick...Even to move around a little bit I

---

[73] Meyers D. The Greatest Male Gymnast Of All Time Eats Just One Meal A Day. DEADSPIN 2017 Sept 27. <https://deadspin.com/the-greatest-male-gymnast-of-all-time-eats-just-one-mea-1818839852>

like to be empty...When I'm empty, I feel like it's easy to move and I'm in a good state."

You may fear that doing exercise before eating will make you extremely ravenous, but research has shown that doing physical activity in a fasted state has little impact on appetite or may even reduce appetite.[74, 75] This occurs simply because ongoing physical and mental activities are primarily fueled by your abundant body energy reserves, not by recent food intake. A typical physical exercise session will expend 500 to 1000 kcal, which is only 0.3% of the energy in stored fat and glycogen, a trivial expenditure of energy reserves. Further, exercise stimulates the release of stored fat and glycogen into the blood, and because this is similar to the post-meal condition, it favors reduced food intake for some time after an intense exercise session.

[74] Rogers PJ, Brunstrom JM, "Appetite and energy balancing," *Physiology & Behavior* 6 April 2016. pii: S0031-9384 (16) 30119-6.

[75] Gonzalez JT, Veasey RC, Rumbold PLS, Stevenson EJ. Breakfast and exercise contingently affect postprandial metabolism and energy balance in physically active males. Br J Nutr 2013 Aug 28;110(4):721-732.

Manufacturers of breakfast foods have claimed that skipping meals will cause poor mental performance, but this has been refuted. In fact, for most people, eating a substantial breakfast tends to impair performance.[76]

Many people notice feeling sleepy after substantial meals, particularly carbohydrate-rich meals, and some take this to be a sign of some physical imbalance or that carbohydrates are harmful. It is neither. This occurs because digesting meals diverts energy away from the central nervous system and stimulates the rest-and-digest parasympathetic nervous system response. Also, if the meal contains substantial carbohydrate, the sudden rise in blood glucose and insulin drives more L-tryptophan into the brain, which increases the production of sleep-inducing melatonin. Thus it is natural and expected to feel sleepy after substantial carbohydrate-rich meals, especially if you are already in the middle of your feeding period (e.g. after lunch). This is why traditional cultures scheduled a siesta after the main mid-day meal.

---

[76] Ibid.

This effect may be reduced if you have fasted sufficiently and done significant physical activity prior to eating the first meal, so that the incoming carbohydrate gets delivered to glycogen stores.

Also, meals high in protein but low in carbohydrate (turkey without the stuffing, potatoes and bread, i.e. a primal food meal) increases blood levels of L-tyrosine and L-phenylalanine, both of which compete with L-tryptophan for transportation across the blood-brain barrier, and these amino acids favor increased brain levels of adrenaline, dopamine, and noradrenaline, which improve alertness and acuity. Hence, combining a high protein, low carbohydrate meal plan with time-restricted feeding favors high mental performance.

9 Implementing Primal Fasting

As already noted, in this manual, fasting means not eating or drinking anything that provides energy (calories). Most people do an absolute fast for some 8-10 hours overnight. To obtain the benefits of absolute fasting discussed above, it is necessary to extend the daily fasting period to about 16-18 hours, or to fast 24 to 36 hours once or twice weekly, or combine these two approaches.

In essence, this means either delaying your break fast, or eliminating an evening meal, or some combination of these two. Its really not complicated, but entails changing habits and riding out any discomfort you may experience as you adjust to the new schedule.

You might feel intimidated by the idea of fasting 16-18 hours and eating only two meals on a daily basis, even more by the suggestion of one or two 20-24 hour fasts each week, but once you actually try it for several weeks, I think you will want to continue indefinitely.

Ground Rules

During your fasting periods you may consume non-caloric beverages including:

- Water (preferably filtered with a solid carbon block filter)
- Herbal teas
- Green or black tea
- Coffee

Without cream or sweeteners.

I recommend avoiding all beverages sweetened with artificial non-caloric sweeteners. Studies show refined sugar and non-caloric sweeteners have addictive properties, making you want more sweets and sweet flavors in your food. In one study, mice given the choice of unlimited access to cocaine, sugar, or saccharine chose sugar or saccharine over cocaine even if they were previously addicted to cocaine.[77] In addition, we have considerable evidence that eating

---

[77] Lenoir M, Serre F, Cantin L, Ahmed SH, "Intense Sweetness Surpasses Cocaine Reward," *PLoS ONE* 2007 ;2(8): e698. doi: 10.1371/ journal.pone.0000698

non-caloric sweeteners stimulate sweets cravings, overeating and weight gain.[78]

One purpose of a fast is to break your addiction to intensely sweetened foods. Generally, limit the use of all non-caloric sweeteners during a fast. I recommend drinking water, herbal tea, black tea, roasted green tea, black coffee, roasted chicory tea, or roasted dandelion tea during your fast.

Extending Your Daily Fast

The easiest way to gain the benefits of fasting lies in limiting yourself to two daily meals and fitting all the meals of any day into a feeding period lasting 6 to 8 hours, thus extending the daily period of continuous fasting to 16 to 18 hours. Here's how to transition to time-restricted feeding:

Step 1: Eliminate snacks

---

[78] Yang Q, "Gain weight by "going diet?" Artificial sweeteners and the neurobiology of sugar cravings: Neuroscience 2010," *The Yale Journal of Biology and Medicine* 2010;83(2):101-108. <http://www.ncbi.nlm.nih.gov/pmc/articles/PMC2892765/?tool>

If you've been eating more than 3 times daily, start by cutting out all of your snacks and reducing to not more than 3 meals daily. At the times you would have eaten a snack or snacks, have a non-caloric beverage. If you have been eating only two or three meals daily, move on to step 2.

Step 2: Identify your optimum daily feeding period

As already noted, from a biological standpoint, a significant and growing body of research indicates that humans and some other mammals sustain better metabolic health when they consume most of their food early in their normal waking period (for humans, daylight hours) rather than late in the day.[79, 80, 81] People assigned to consuming the bulk of their food

---

[79] Jakubowicz D, Barnea M, et al., "Effects of caloric intake timing on insulin resistance and hyperandrogenism in lean women with polycystic ovary syndrome," *Clinical Science* 2013 Nov 01;125(9): 423-432. <http://www.clinsci.org/content/125/9/423.long>

[80] Morgan LM, Shi J-W, et al., "Effect of meal timing and glycaemic index on glucose control and insulin secretion in healthy volunteers," *Br J Nutr* 2012;108:1286-1291.

[81] Jakubowicz D, Barnea M, et al., "High Caloric intake at breakfast vs. dinner differentially influences weight loss of overweight and obese women," *Obesity* 2013 Dec;21(12);2504-2512. <http://onlinelibrary.wiley.com/doi/10.1002/oby.20460/full>

early in the day showed less hunger, greater satiety, lower body fat mass, smaller waist circumference, and lower serum glucose, triglycerides, and insulin levels than those who consumed the bulk of their food late in the day.[82] People who eat late rather than early meals have a higher propensity to gain weight and more difficulty losing it.[83] This occurs because eating during the early part of the day synchronizes with circadian cycles of hormones and organ functions.[84]

In another study, complaints of daytime hunger were common among individuals who participated in an experiment where they consumed all their food in one 4-hour long evening meal.[85]

---

[82] Ibid.

[83] Garaulet M, Gómez-Abellán P, "Timing of food intake and obesity: A novel association," *Physiology & Behavior* 2014 Jul; 134:44-50. <http://www.tradewindsports.net/wp-content/uploads/2014/03/Nutrient-Timing-and-Obesity-2014.pdf>

[84] Ibid..

[85] Stote KS, Baer DJ, Spears K, et al., "A controlled trial of reduced meal frequency without caloric restriction in healthy, normal-weight, middle-aged adults," The Am J Clin Nutr 2007;85(4):981-988. <http://www.ncbi.nlm.nih.gov/pmc/articles/PMC2645638/>

Chinese medicine maintains that all organs have circadian variations in functions. According to Chinese medical theory, the stomach is most receptive to food and most capable of efficient digestion in the hours 7-9 A.M. and weakest in the hours 7-9 P.M.. Biomedical research has confirmed that the stomach empties about 50% more quickly after a meal taken at 8 A.M. compared to a meal taken at 8 P.M.,[86] so food stagnation, indigestion and acid reflux may occur when large meals are taken in the evening rather than the morning. This may also contribute to constipation, as stagnation in the stomach will often impair intestinal peristalsis.

An earlier feeding schedule supports deep sleep as well. Due to the fact that the stomach empties more slowly in the evening, taking large meals within three hours of going to sleep can result in restless, dream-filled, unsatisfying sleep. For most people, sleep is sounder when the stomach has emptied by the time one goes to sleep. If you suffer from sleep disturbance, you may want to try having your last large meal

[86] Goo RH, Moore JG, et al., "Circadian Variation in Gastric Emptying of Meals in Humans," *Gastroenterology* 1987;93:515-8. <http://www.gastrojournal.org/article/0016-5085(87)90913-9/pdf>

finished five or six hours before you go to bed. This will usually result in having an appetite for breaking fast earlier in the next day.

Many people report having no appetite in the early morning. I have found that people who have no appetite before noon generally have a habit of eating large meals late in the day. Since late meals are digested inefficiently, you may feel food sitting in your gut when you awaken in the morning. The remedy is quite simple. If one skips or minimizes the last meal of the day, one will generally have a stronger appetite early in the day.

As already noted, some proportion of Seventh Day Adventists eat two meals, generally morning and noon, and SDAs have lower risks of chronic diseases and have a greater healthy life expectancy than the average American.[87] Also, for centuries, many Buddhists have followed the traditional discipline to only eat food in the

---

[87] Kelly CJ, "A controlled trial of reduced meal frequency without caloric restriction in healthy, normal-weight, middle-aged adults," *Am J Clin Nutr* 2007 Oct; 86(4): 1254-1255. <http://ajcn.nutrition.org/content/86/4/1254.2.long>

hours between dawn and noon, and fast until dawn after their mid-day meal.

Tracy and I roughly follow this pattern. We are generally up and about, doing meditation, writing, household chores, mobility training, or strength training, for 2-4 hours before we begin to feel noticeable hunger. After spending 2 to 4 hours doing these various tasks, we usually break fast sometime between 9 and 10 A.M.. Between 10 A.M. and 2 P.M., we may have a smaller snack. Then we eat our second meal around 2-3 P.M. and usually finish by 4-6 P.M.. After the second main meal we generally don't feel hungry until about 8 or 10 A.M. the next day, so we find it relatively easy to fast for 16-18 hours daily with very little time spent feeling hunger.

If you eat a late breakfast and a main mid-afternoon meal, you will likely feel satisfied all day, through the evening, and spend the longest part of your daily fast asleep. Then, when you awaken, your body will have already shifted overnight into metabolism supported by energy stores (fat and glycogen), which will blunt your morning appetite. Thus you will be able to engage in physical and/or mentally challenging activities for at least a couple of hours before you will feel a strong desire to eat. If you wait to eat until later in the day, hunger will arise, and it can be hard to concentrate on other tasks when you feel hungry. We prefer getting our hunger satisfied first, which then frees our attention for our other activities.

While many people think of the evening as the best time for the family to share a meal, morning may present an even better opportunity. Children of modern families typically have after-school activities that prevent the family from all being together for an evening meal at the same time. Father or mother may be involved in long hours or overtime at work, meetings, chauffeuring children to their activities, volunteering, night school, exercise, or other business. It is often easier for a family to eat together in the morning, before the members disperse in different directions (school, work, etc.). Having a substantial home-cooked meal early in the day also ensures that everyone starts the day off on the right nutritional foot, well-satisfied so less prone to grabbing junk food during the day.

On the other hand, as noted in the previous chapter, in the only published research on time-restricted feeding in strength athletes, the subjects started their eating window at 1 p.m. and continued to 9 p.m., with good body composition and metabolic results.[88] Even if eating earlier in the day gives the *best* results, this study suggests that you can still get *good* results by eating in a window starting in the early afternoon and ending by 9 p.m..

Since the evidence indicates that you might get the best health and fitness results by eating more food between morning and mid-day and little or none in the evening, I strongly urge you to give this approach a trial if your schedule permits. However, your schedule may not permit this and your experience with morning vs. afternoon or evening eating may vary. If you find that it is more enjoyable or practical for you to have your meal window in the later part of the day, you can still

---

[88] Moro T, Tinsley G, Bianco A, et al.. Effects of eight weeks of time-restricted feeding (16/8) on basal metabolism, maximal strength, body composition, inflammation, and cardiovascular risk factors in resistance-trained males. J Translational Med 2016 October 13;14:290. <https://translational-medicine.biomedcentral.com/articles/10.1186/s12967-016-1044-0>

get the benefits of periodic fasting. Just adhere to the principle of fasting about 16 hours (give or take an hour) every day.

Timing exercise

When you increase your daily fasting period, you will eat larger meals during your eating window and these will take several hours to digest. If you don't do your intense physical training at the end of your fasting period, you will want to do it a couple of hours after any large meal you eat. We prefer doing our regular resistance and mobility training in the morning before eating, partly because it is more comfortable on an empty stomach, partly because this prevents us from missing training sessions due to getting involved in other tasks during the day, and partly because training before breaking fast may have other benefits.

Research suggests that training hard before breaking the overnight fast results in greater appetite control and reductions of body fat.[89] Morning aerobic exercise may induce greater reductions of blood pressure and more time spent in deep sleep compared to afternoon training.[90]

You may however find that you prefer doing intense training in the afternoon or evening. If so, finishing your meals in the late afternoon may still be the best solution. If you don't eat in the evening, this will give you time to exercise, several hours after finishing your meal. Then you can fast until the next morning. However, if you prefer to wait to break fast until about mid-day, then you may have opportunity to train in the late-afternoon after a mid-afternoon snack, and finish the day with a substantial supper after training.

Step 3: Reduce to two main meals

---

[89] Gonzalez JT, Veasey RC, Rumbold PLS, Stevenson EJ. Breakfast and exercise contingently affect postprandial metabolism and energy balance in physically active males. Br J Nutr 2013 Aug 28;110(4):721-732.

[90] Fairbrother K, Cartner B, Alley JR, et al. Effects of exercise timing on sleep architecture and nocturnal blood pressure in prehypertensives. *Vascular Health and Risk Management.* 2014;10:691-698. doi:10.2147/VHRM.S73688.

Some evidence suggests that eating two meals daily produces a better metabolic condition than either one or three meals. Animals fed two early meals (breakfast and mid-day) had less body weight and fat gain than those fed either three meals or two late meals, but both groups fed only two meals fared better in some metabolic respects than the group fed three meals.[91]

Another study found that animals fed a large breakfast with a smaller supper (two meals daily) fared better than those fed the same amount and type of food in one single daily meal (breakfast only).[92] Those on one meal experienced an increase in body weight gain, elevated blood levels of insulin and leptin, a disturbance of the circadian expression of the Clock gene, and a reduction of gene expression associated with fat oxidation (ß-oxidation) in both fat cells and the liver, in comparison to those eating two meals daily.

[91] Wu T, Sun L, ZhuGe F, et al., "Differential Roles of Breakfast and Supper in Rats of a Daily Three-Meal Schedule Upon Circadian Regulation and Physiology," *Chronobiology International* 2011 Nov 14;28(10):890-903.

[92] Fuse Y, et al., 2012. Op. cit. (note 29).

Humans may respond a little differently to a one-evening-meal-a-day plan. As already noted, an 8 week long human study compared the effects of eating all caloric requirements in just one as opposed to the conventional three meals per day.[93] In contrast to the just-discussed rodent study, this study found that the people assigned to fasting 20 hours daily, then eating all of their caloric requirements in only 1 evening meal each day lost an average of 1.4 kg (3 lb.) body mass and 2.1 kg (4.6 lb.) fat mass over the eight weeks. However, these people did report experiencing increased daytime hunger, which is not reported by people assigned to eat most of their calories early in the day.

Thus, two meals daily might be more sustainable than one meal daily, and it might also produce better health results than either one or three. (Limiting oneself to only one meal on one or two days per week or month is different because doing this infrequently does not

---

[93] Stote KS, Raer DJ, Spears K, et al, "A controlled trial of reduced meal frequency without caloric restriction in healthy, normal-weight, middle-aged adults," *Am J Clin Nutr* 2007;85(4):981-988. <http://www.ncbi.nlm.nih.gov/pmc/articles/PMC2645638/>

enforce metabolic adaptations to one meal daily; see below.)

If you feel intimidated by the two-meal plan, one way to gradually get adjusted to longer daily fasting involves doing it one day of your first week of implementation, then add one day each week, so that by the end of 7 weeks you have completely adapted your daily schedule to have a 16-18 hour fast each day. Once you finish this process, if desired you can gradually reduce your eating window from 8 hours to 4-6 hours in the same fashion. The following table illustrates the process I have suggested.

Week	Sun.	Mon.	Tues.	Wed.	Thur.	Fri.	Sat.
Table 9.1: A possible process for gradually adapting to daily fasting intervals of 16 hours or more.							
1	*Fast 16+hrs, eat 2 meals*	Fast 12 hrs —3 meals	Fast 12 hrs –3 meals	Fast 12 hrs –3 meals	Fast 12 hrs – 3 meals	Fast 12 hrs – 3 meals	Fast 12 hrs – 3 meals
2	*Fast 16+hrs, eat 2 meals*	*Fast 16+hrs, eat 2 meals*	Fast 12 hrs—3 meals	Fast 12 hrs—3 meals	Fast 12 hrs—3 meals	Fast 12 hrs—3 meals	Fast 12 hrs—3 meals

3	Fast 16+hrs, eat 2 meals	Fast 16+hrs, eat 2 meals	Fast 16+hrs, eat 2 meals	Fast 12 hrs—3 meals	Fast 12 hrs—3 meals	Fast 12 hrs—3 meals	Fast 12 hrs—3 meals
4	Fast 16+hrs, eat 2 meals	Fast 16+hrs, eat 2 meals	Fast 16+hrs, eat 2 meals	Fast 16+hrs, eat 2 meals	Fast 12 hrs—3 meals	Fast 12 hrs—3 meals	Fast 12 hrs—3 meals
5	Fast 16+hrs, eat 2 meals	Fast 16+hrs, eat 2 meals	Fast 16+hrs, eat 2 meals	Fast 16+hrs, eat 2 meals	Fast 16+hrs, eat 2 meals	Fast 12 hrs—3 meals	Fast 12 hrs—3 meals
6	Fast 16+hrs, eat 2 meals	Fast 16+hrs, eat 2 meals	Fast 16+hrs, eat 2 meals	Fast 16+hrs, eat 2 meals	Fast 16+hrs, eat 2 meals	Fast 16+hrs, eat 2 meals	Fast 12 hrs—3 meals
7	Fast 16+hrs, eat 2 meals	Fast 16+hrs, eat 2 meals	Fast 16+hrs, eat 2 meals	Fast 16+hrs, eat 2 meals	Fast 16+hrs, eat 2 meals	Fast 16+hrs, eat 2 meals	Fast 16+hrs, eat 2 meals

Eat your two daily meals within an 8 hour period or less. For example, eat breakfast between 7 and 10 a.m. and start your last meal 3 to 6 hours after you finish breakfast. Or, eat breakfast at mid-day and finish your last meal 6 hours later. In this way you can arrange a 16 to 20 hour fast each day.

Remember, on days when you have only 2 meals, you can eat to satisfaction of whole foods at both of those meals. Fasting regularly generally improves your selection of foods. After you fast 16 or more hours, you will generally prefer healthy, substantial foods, not junk.

How I Eased Into Time-Restricted Feeding

Many years ago, when I first started daily extended fasting, I first eliminated my fourth daily feeding, which was an evening snack about 7 P.M.. This made me feel hungrier in the morning, so I started increasing the caloric content of my breakfast.

By eating a larger breakfast I was able to delay my second meal to a little later time. Then I just made the second meal large enough to keep me satisfied through the evening, and easily eliminated what had been the third meal of the day.

That left me with two meals: my breakfast, usually taken between 8 and 10 A.M., and my supper, usually started between 2 and 3 P.M., or when really hungry from hard training I will have a snack around 1 or 2 P.M. and then eat a large meal about 4 or 5 P.M..

Weekly Fasts

Although based on the research cited above I don't consider this optimal, some people may prefer to eat a normal 3 meals daily on most days, but fast for 20-24 hours once or twice weekly. This is better than not fasting at all. Others may want to combine daily ~16-18 hour fasts with longer 20-24 hour fasts once or twice weekly.

Fasting 24 hours once or twice weekly is a simple (but not necessarily easy) way to reduce your total energy intake to achieve fat loss, without having to endure hunger every day. Removing one or two meals from one day will reduce your calorie intake by 1000-2000 calories; done twice weekly you will create a caloric deficit that will result in a loss of one-half to one pound of fat weekly.

To fast 24 hours, abstain from food from the last meal of one day to the same time the next day. Based on personal experience and the data showing that large morning meals produce a greater satiety and less hunger sensation than skipping early meals to only eat a late meal, I would recommend the 24 hour fast be accomplished by eating a substantial early (8-10 A.M.) breakfast, then fasting 24 hours until the same time the next morning. If you finish breakfast at 10 A.M. you would fast until 10 A.M. the next day, at which time you would have a substantial breakfast. Alternatively, you can fast from evening to evening – e.g. from 6 P.M. Monday to 6 P.M. Tuesday – although I think that, due to daytime hunger, you will find this will be much more challenging than fasting from morning to morning.

To fast 36 hours on occasion, abstain from food from the last meal of one day to the morning two days later; for example, from 6 P.M. Friday evening to 6 A.M. Sunday morning.

Limiting oneself to only one meal daily only once or twice weekly will not train the body to increase fat storage and reduce fat oxidation because the 24 hour fasts occur infrequently and interrupted by 3-6 days of regular food intake.

A schedule with 14-hr fasts daily and one 24-hr fast in a week could look like this:

Day	Feeding	Fasting
1	8 A.M. – 6 P.M.	6 P.M. D1 – 8 A.M. D2
2	8 A.M. – 6 P.M.	6 P.M. D2 – 8 A.M. D3
3	8 A.M. – 6 P.M.	6 P.M. D3 – 8 A.M. D4
4	8 A.M. – 6 P.M.	6 P.M. D4 – 8 A.M. D5
5	8 A.M. – 6 P.M.	9 A.M. D5 – 9 A.M. D6
6 Fast to 9 A.M.	9 A.M. – 6 P.M.	6 P.M. D6 – 8 A.M. D7
7	8 A.M. – 6 P.M.	6 P.M. D7 – 8 A.M. D8

A schedule with two 24-hr fasts in a week could look like this:

Day	Feeding	Fasting
1	8 A.M. – 6 P.M.	6 P.M. D1 – 8 A.M. D2
2	8 A.M. – 9 A.M.	9 A.M. D2 – 9 P.M. D3
3 Fast to 9 A.M.	9 A.M. – 6 P.M.	6 P.M. D3 – 8 A.M. D4
4	8 A.M. – 6 P.M.	6 P.M. D4 – 8 A.M. D5
5	8 A.M. – 9 A.M.	9 A.M. D5 – 9 P.M. D6
6 Fast to 9 A.M.	9 A.M. – 6 P.M.	6 P.M. D6 – 8 A.M. D7
7	8 A.M. – 6 P.M.	6 P.M. D7 – 8 A.M. D8

You can adjust the daily feeding window and fasting period to your preference. For example, you could restrict your daily feeding window to 8 A.M. – 4 P.M. so that you fast 16 hours daily *and* once or twice weekly, extend that fast to 24 hours.

Primal fasting

All natural phenomena fluctuate in cycles. Civilized people tend to follow schedules, enact habits, or pursue goals that may lead to reduced awareness of the body's natural cycles. Without adequate awareness of or respect for body rhythms, one might eat out of habit, or because one has a goal (e.g. to gain muscle), in spite of a lack of hunger or appetite. Unlike non-human animals, humans can get into trouble because we are prone to follow ideology rather than biology.

Chinese medical theory values prevention of disease over cure. It is best to take care of imbalances when they are small – nip them in the bud, as a European sage would say – than to exert heroic efforts after leaving something go until it becomes a crisis. In the *Yellow Emperor's Classic of Internal Medicine,* the Emperor's chief physician, Qi Bo explains:

> Those who wait to treat disease until it has already arisen are like those who wait until they are thirsty to dig a well, or wait until they are in battle to forge weapons. Are not these actions too late?

Disease prevention hinges on knowing the early signs heralding its emergence. One of the signs of impending illness is a decline in appetite. One will lack appetite when the body needs to invest energy in activities other than digesting foods, such as cleaning metabolic wastes or excess nutrients out of cells or tissues, or fighting off an invader (virus, bacteria). Thus, if one has a sense of fatigue and a loss of appetite, one may be on the verge of acute illness. If one does the right thing at the right time, one can avert trouble.

Adhering to this principle, I practice extended fasting when dictated by fluctuations in my appetite and energy levels. Whenever I feel unusual fatigue and a disinterest in food accompanying a feeling of prolonged fullness (simple indigestion) after a meal, I embark on a fast and spend more time in relaxing activities and sleep until my appetite returns full force. Usually it will return after about 24 hours of fasting, but sometimes I need two days with 24 hours of fasting, or one 36 hour fast. After the fast I feel rejuvenated.

10 Fasting For Fat Loss

In order to lose body fat, you absolutely must create and sustain a negative fat balance and to do this you need to create and sustain a hormonal environment that favors fat expenditure over fat storage.

Most often people try to cut down on the size of meals, resulting in meal-by-meal calorie counting. This has the drawback of increasing the amount of attention you have to give to planning meals and thinking about what and how much you will eat, which may actually have the undesired effect of stimulating appetite. In addition, if your small meals contain any significant carbohydrate, they will produce a rise in blood insulin levels, which favors fat storage and terminates fat expenditure. Further, small meals can tease you, in that you get a little to eat, but not enough to feel satisfied in the moment. This teasing can lead you to eat more when you are trying to eat less.

It is much simpler to just skip some meals, which reduces your contact with food and limits your eating opportunities. Further, when you go longer without eating, you can eat to satisfaction, and get all the pleasure of eating at the meals you do eat, but still maintain a fat and energy deficit. Finally, going longer periods between meals results in lower insulin and higher glucagon levels, which favors fat burning over fat storage.

Some authors suggest that skipping meals will lead you to overeat at later meals. I believed this myself at one time, but research shows that although people who are assigned to delay eating until noon-time do eat a little more at their mid-day meal than they would if they hadn't delayed breakfast, they do not end up eating more calories than they would normally eat at snacks and supper, and they end up with an overall lower caloric intake which will result in fat loss.[94] As discussed in chapter 9, research indicates that skipping evening meals might produce greater fat loss and health benefits than avoiding eating early in the day. However, as always, the best choice for you is the one that you can and will carry out.

---

[94] Rogers PJ, Brunstrom JM, "Appetite and energy balancing," *Physiology & Behavior* 6 April 2016. pii: S0031-9384 (16) 30119-6.

Many people sabotage their ability to get lean through unrealistic expectations. Human metabolism has many rate-limited processes. As already mentioned, humans evolved in an environment where they had to expend considerable energy to acquire adequate food from a habitat wherein food resources were relatively limited. Any human ancestor who lost fat rapidly during lean seasons would have perished. Ancestors who burned off fat reserves very slowly were more likely to survive tight times and leave healthy children.

Consequently, the human body burns fat reserves conservatively. Research has shown that the maximum rate of fat loss is about 30 kcal per pound of excess body fat per day.[95] This means that you should not restrict your weekly food energy intake any more than 210 kcal per pound of fat you want to lose. If you restrict your food energy intake more than that, you will automatically lose lean body mass you do not want to lose.

---

[95] Alpert SS, "A limit on the energy transfer rate from the human fat store in hypophagia," *J Theor Biol* 2005 Mar 7;233(1):1-13.

This has several implications. First, as you become leaner, your rate of fat loss declines. Second, as you become leaner, you must gradually adjust your energy intake (per pound of body mass) upward to prevent loss of lean mass (Table 10.1).

Table 10.1: Maximum daily kcal reduction and rate of fat loss possible without loss of lean mass.			
Desired fat loss (lb.)	Maximum daily fat kcal deficit	Maximum weekly weight loss (lb.)	*Minimum* time required to lose (days)
10	300	0.6	117
20	600	1.2	156
30	900	1.8	174
40	1200	2.4	187
50	1500	3	194

If you want to lose body fat as fast as possible, follow these guidelines:

1. Eat a high protein ancestral diet (see Chapter 12). High protein intake increases satiety and

spontaneously reduces total energy intake.[96, 97] Protein intake also raises levels of glucagon, the main hormone that stimulates fat burning. Increase your protein intake to at least 1 gram per pound of lean body mass. For example, if your desired weight is 160 pounds, consume 160 grams of protein daily. If you have plenty of body fat to burn, you can consume as much as 40-50% of your dietary calories from protein.

2. Keep your fat intake below your fat oxidation rate, which is about 60% of total energy expenditure. The less food fat you consume, the more body fat you will burn. Consume no more than 50%, and as low as 30% of your calories from fat. Eat any cut of meat that supplies at least as many protein calories as fat calories. Eggs are ideal for fat loss because they are about 50% protein calories and 50% fat calories. Limit concentrated free fats and oils, including butter, cream, lard, suet, and all plant-

---

[96] Martens EA, Lemmens SG, Westerterp-Plantenga MS. Protein leverage affects energy intake of high-protein diets in humans. Am J Clin Nutr 2013 Jan;(97(1):86-93. <http://ajcn.nutrition.org/content/97/1/86.full>

[97] Felton AM, Felton A, Raubenheimer D, et al.. Protein content of diets dictates the daily energy intake of a free-ranging primate. Behavioral Ecology. doi:10.1093/beheco/arp021.

based oils. Limit nuts and seeds to no more than 2 ounces per day for men, and 1 ounce per day for women.

3. To reduce your insulin exposure, restrict your carbohydrate intake to no more than 100 g per day, preferably no more than 75 g per day. Achieve this by avoiding plant foods or limiting your plant food intake to only fibrous, brightly colored plant foods, such as green vegetables, onion family vegetables, mushrooms, berries, and nuts. Note, some people may need to limit carbohydrates or plant foods even more to achieve desired results. You may need to adopt a fully carnivorous diet (little or no plant foods) to achieve your goals.

4. To further reduce insulin exposure, fast 16 to 18 hours every day, reduce the number of times you eat in a day to two – preferably breakfast and mid-day – and consider eating only one meal and fasting 20-24 hours on 1 or 2 days each week.

11 Fasting For Building Muscle

Intermittent fasting can help you gain muscle and strength without putting on unwanted fat if you have a regular program of high intensity, progressive resistance strength training and understand how to appropriately manage your food intake to ensure adequate energy and protein intake during your feeding windows.

You must regularly perform progressive resistance training in order to build or retain muscle. The body will not build new muscle tissue or maintain the muscle it already has unless it is required to cope with the type of activity it regularly encounters. Only progressive resistance training that places a demand on muscle strength – not endurance – can stimulate muscle gains.

Fasting favors lean gains

Fasting 16-18 hours daily trains your body to have greater efficiency at utilizing nutrients during your feeding periods. During absolute fasting, the body shifts into a hormonal condition aimed at preserving muscle while burning fat, because in ancient times, one would need to have the muscle to successfully hunt during fasting periods and therefore survive the fast. As discussed already, prolonging your daily fasting period favors higher levels of growth hormone production, and growth hormone promotes both fat loss and muscle growth. Once you eat, this muscle preservation system directs the nutrients you consume to the muscular system to prepare for the next fast and food quest.

As previously noted, an 8 week long human study compared the effects of eating all caloric requirements in just one as opposed to the conventional three meals per day.[98] This study found that the people assigned to fasting 20 hours daily, then eating all of their caloric requirements in only 1 evening meal each day lost an average of 1.4 kg (3 lb.) body mass and 2.1 kg (4.6 lb.) fat mass over the eight weeks, which means that they gained an average of 1.6 lb. lean mass over the study period, with no change in energy intake or exercise

---

[98] Stote KS, Baer DJ, Spears K, et al, "A controlled trial of reduced meal frequency without caloric restriction in healthy, normal-weight, middle-aged adults," *Am J Clin Nutr* 2007;85(4):981-988. <http://www.ncbi.nlm.nih.gov/pmc/articles/PMC2645638/>

habits. If not experimental error, this increase in lean mass may have resulted from increased growth hormone output that occurs during fasting. However, the authors did not determine whether this apparent increase in lean mass consisted of water, glycogen, muscle, organ tissue, or bone, or some combination. Nevertheless, this report indicates that reducing meal frequency does not lead to loss of lean mass, and may promote lean mass gains.

As previously mentioned, a study of 8 weeks of daily time-restricted feeding (16 hours fasting/8 hour feeding) compared to conventional feeding schedule (11 hours fasting/13 hours feeding) in subjects engaged in resistance training thrice weekly found that the TRF group showed decreases in fat mass, blood glucose, insulin, triglycerides, and markers of inflammation, while simultaneously increasing in lean mass, arm and thigh cross-sectional area, bench press and leg press 1-RM.[99]

---

[99] Moro T, Tinsley G, Bianco A, et al.. Effects of eight weeks of time-restricted feeding (16/8) on basal metabolism, maximal strength, body composition, inflammation, and cardiovascular risk factors in resistance trained males. J Trans Med 2016 Oct 13;14:290. <https://translational-medicine.biomedcentral.com/articles/10.1186/s12967-016-1044-0>

Feasting favors fat gains

Contrary to common belief, it is not necessary nor beneficial to *overeat* in order to build muscle. If you have at least 10% body fat, you have plenty of energy reserves to draw upon for fueling muscle growth that occurs after high intensity training sessions. Further, if you sustain an *excess* caloric intake and high insulin level (due to high carbohydrate intake) for more than a few days in a row, the majority of the excess energy you consume ends up stored as body fat, not muscle mass. The key here is to understand what constitutes an excess energy intake or overeating.

Studies show that deliberate overeating does result in some apparent lean mass gain, but it also favors fat gain over time. In one study, subjects who overate 1200-1600 kcal daily gained 4 pounds of lean mass and 4.7 pounds of fat over the course of 21 days.[100] Thus, only about 46% of weight gained by overeating (without concurrent resistance exercise) consisted of

---

[100] Forbes GB, Brown MR, Welle SL, Underwood LE, "Hormonal response to overfeeding," *Am J Clin Nutr* 1989;49:608-11.

non-fat mass. However, while some of this lean gain could have been muscle the authors did not determine exactly what proportion of the lean gains obtained by overeating consists of increases in intestinal contents, retention of water and storage of glycogen, as opposed to contractile muscle tissue.

Thus the fact that you gain weight and some lean mass during overeating does not indicate that overeating itself can add muscle mass to the body. If overeating effectively promoted muscle growth, one could gain muscle simply by overeating to gain both fat and muscle, then dieting to lose the fat and expose the muscle. Ask yourself: When overweight people reduce their fat mass by diet, do we find them now sporting an unusually muscular physique? We all know this does not happen.

In fact, excess caloric intake does not promote muscle gains. The body only adds muscle tissue if it must do so to adapt to the types of force production demands regularly imposed upon it.

Moreover, proper training to stimulate muscle growth will increase one's hunger if the combination of food intake and energy available from body fat stores does not satisfy the increased energy demands. If in response to a training-stimulated increased appetite you spontaneously (and appropriately) consume enough food to satisfy your hunger and meet the energy demands of training and muscle growth, you will not be overeating – which is defined as consuming more calories than you need – but will be eating just what Nature demands to maintain energy balance.

Simply put, excess food intake always leads to fat gain, not muscle gain; while eating an increased amount of food to satisfy a training-stimulated increase in hunger is not overeating. If you eat animal protein and fat, and little carbohydrate, as dictated by your hunger, you can expect to gain muscle and very little fat. If you eat more than your hunger dictates, expect to gain fat, especially if you choose plant foods rich in carbohydrate.

Long-term overeating (i.e. consuming more food than needed to satisfy your hunger and body demands) in order to "bulk up" may actually reduce your capacity to gain muscle, because it increases fat gain and insulin resistance within days,[101] and obesity and insulin resistance are both associated with increased myostatin expression.[102] Myostatin suppresses muscle growth and insulin resistance impedes protein synthesis. Resistance exercise, aerobic exercise, and body fat loss through caloric restriction all independently reduce expression of myostatin.[103] Thus, deliberate overeating (again, eating more than your hunger dictates), particularly of carbohydrate-rich foods, actually counteracts the myostatin-reducing (muscle-building) effects of resistance exercise, while eating only whatever additional food you need to

---

[101] Boden G, Homko C, Barrero CA, et al., "Excessive caloric intake acutely causes oxidative stress, GLUT4 carbonylation, and insulin resistance in healthy men," *Sci Transl Med.* 2015;7(304).

[102] Allen DL, Hittel DS, McPherron AC, "Expression and Function of Myostatin in Obesity, Diabetes, and Exercise Adaptation," *Medicine and science in sports and exercise.* 2011;43(10): 1828-1835. doi:10.1249/MSS.0b013e3182178bb4. <https://www.ncbi.nlm.nih.gov/pmc/articles/PMC3192366/>

[103] Ryan AS, Li G, Blumenthal JB, Ortmeyer HK, "Aerobic Exercise+Weight Loss Decreases Skeletal Muscle Myostatin Expression and Improves Insulin Sensitivity in Older Adults," *Obesity (Silver Spring, Md).* 2013;21(7):1350-1356. doi:10.1002/oby.20216.
<https://www.ncbi.nlm.nih.gov/pmc/articles/PMC3742694/>

satisfy your training-stimulated hunger probably increases your ability to gain muscle by reducing expression of myostatin.

Most people in industrialized populations already have more than enough excess calories stored on their bodies in the form of fat to support abundant muscle growth. For example, a 140 pound male at 10% body fat carries 14 pounds of fat. About half of that is essential fat that can't be used for energy, so 7 pounds of his body fat is available for energy reserves and provides 24,500 kcalories. A pound of muscle itself is 70% water, and about 30% protein, so it represents the storage of only 136 g of protein and 550 kcal. Hence, a man carrying just 7 pounds of non-essential fat has energy reserves equivalent to the caloric value of nearly 45 pounds of muscle!

Average American men and women have about 28 and 40% body fat, respectively. American men and women with *normal* Body Mass Indices (< 25) have an average body fat of 23 and 34%.[104] Thus, most Americans, including those who may appear lean to the untrained observer, have plenty of excess energy available on their bodies to fuel muscle growth. They do not need to increase their caloric intake for this purpose.

Table 11.1: Body Fat Percentage Categories		
Category	**Women**	**Men**
Athletes	14-20%	6-13%
Fitness	21-24%	14-17%
Average	25-31%	18-24%
Obese	32%+	25%+

How fast can you gain muscle?

Many people try overeating to boost their rate of muscle growth because they are impatient and mistakenly believe that typical trainees can gain muscle at rapid rates, such as 1-2 pounds of muscle per week. (Often they are also using ineffective training

104 St-Onge M-P, "Are Normal-Weight Americans Over-Fat?," Obesity (Silver Spring, Md). 2010;18(11):10.1038/oby.2010.103. doi:10.1038/oby.2010.103. <http://www.ncbi.nlm.nih.gov/pmc/articles/PMC3837418/#R1>

methods that don't stimulate a spontaneous anabolic response.) Research shows that typical novices to progressive resistance training will only gain on average 1-2 pounds of muscle *per month* – that's only one-quarter to one-half pound of muscle per week – with a wide variation between individuals. As one passes the novice stage, the rate of gain tapers considerably as the rate of strength gains slows down and the quest to gain muscle requires more patience and persistence over a long term.[105, 106]

Consider that if you did gain one pound of muscle per week, this would amount to 52 pounds of gain in a year. That would transform the typical 5'10" tall, 154 pound male into a 206 pound individual comparable to an elite bodybuilder. Yet not even elite bodybuilders – who are all of relatively rare genetic stock – gain muscle at this rate.

---

[105] Pilon B, *How Much Protein?* (Strength Works, 2008-2009): 39.

[106] Cureton KJ, et al., "Muscle hypertrophy in men and women," *Medicine and Science in Sports and Exercise* 1988; 20(4): 338-344.

To illustrate: Over his 15 year career, 9-time Mr. Olympia Dorian Yates, a genetically gifted and drug-assisted bodybuilder, gained a total of 70 pounds, an average gain of less than 5 pounds per year. Yates gained more per year in the earlier stages and less later, but this illustrates how difficult it is to gain muscular body mass, even for the genetically gifted. In short, if you were to gain an average of 5 pounds of muscle annually – less than half a pound of muscle per month – over several years you would be matching the average rate of muscle gain found in elite bodybuilders who use anabolic steroids.

Novices can *expect* to gain 10-20 pounds during their first year of proper progressive resistance training, 5-10 pounds in the second year, 2-5 pounds in the third and perhaps fourth year, and 1-2 pounds per year thereafter. Individuals vary and some may gain more and some less than the average. If you gain more than these amounts, consider yourself more gifted than average.

Therefore, in reality most people only need *at most* 550-1100 extra kcalories and 136-272 extra grams of protein *per month* – that's only 20-40 kcalories and 5-9 g protein per day – to sustain genetically typical rates of muscle growth. If you want to add 25-50 pounds of muscle to your body without anabolic drug assistance, count on taking 3-4 years or more to accomplish it unless you are genetically gifted with unusually low myostatin levels.

To reiterate, muscle only grows in response to an imposed demand for an increase in strength (force production capacity), so the most important thing for muscle gain is *progressive* resistance exercise. That means consistent, persistent training that involves a sustainable, gradual significant increase in the resistance against which you exert your force. Any change in muscle mass produced by altering what, when, or how much you eat is of minor significance in comparison to adaptation to progressive resistance exercise.

Proper training means using a program of progressive resistance on heavy compound movements for the major muscle groups, such that will allow large increases in load over time, including:

Table 11.2: Best exercises for the major muscle groups

Muscle groups	Proper exercises
Hips, quadriceps, lower back	Squats
Hamstrings, lower back	Back extension, leg curls
Calves	Standing rise on toes
Upper back, biceps, forearms	Chin ups, rows
Chest, triceps	Parallel bar dips, flat bench press
Shoulders, triceps	Overhead press

Each training session should contain one or two exercises for each major muscle group. For a very simple and effective example:

Routine A:

Squats

Rowing (inverted, barbell, or dumbbell)

Dips, push ups, or bench press

Leg curls

Rise on toes

Sit-up or plank variation

<u>Routine B:</u>

Squats

Chin ups

Overhead press

Back extension

Rise on toes

Side bend or arch up variation

You should train 2-3 times per week, alternating these two routines, and progress the resistance as often as possible. Muscle grows to meet force demands, so you must incrementally increase the weight you move *in good form* in order to stimulate muscle to grow.

The most common mistake is to attempt to increase the resistance used in too large increments, such as 5 or 10 pounds, because most gyms do not have smaller plates for smaller increments. You will need to invest in small weight plates (1/4 and 1/2 pound) so that you can increase the weights you use by as little as 1/2 to 1 pound on at least a weekly basis.

Many people also expect relatively small increases in strength to produce large increases in muscle mass. To gain 40 pounds of muscle, a male trainee starting at about 150 pounds will need to progress to the ability to perform at least 8 repetitions with about 315 pounds in the squat, and at least 6 repetitions with 250 pounds in the full range dips, bench press or rowing, 200 pounds in the overhead press, and bodyweight plus 50 percent (e.g. 170 pounds bodyweight plus 85 pounds additional) in the chin up. In increments, you will need to gain strength (measured in pounds added to the resistance) on major lifts much faster than you gain body mass, in approximately the ratios shown in Table 11.3:[107]

Table 11.3: Approximate strength gains needed per pound of muscle mass increase	
Exercise	Strength gain: muscle gain ratio
Squat	5-6:1
Dips or bench press	4:1

---

[107] These ratios are similar to but higher than those proposed by Martin Berkhan of www.leangains.com. I calculated them by taking the differences between typical early intermediate and advanced strength levels in major movements and dividing those by a projected 40 pound gain of lean mass. For example, the squat: (315-135)÷40=4.5. Rounded to at least 5 pounds gain on the squat for every pound of bodyweight gain.

Table 11.3: Approximate strength gains needed per pound of muscle mass increase

Exercise	Strength gain: muscle gain ratio
Chin ups or rows	4:1

These ratios mean that, after you have achieved neurological adaptation to the movements (no longer a novice), in order to acquire one pound of additional muscle mass, you will need to increase your training loads by *at least* 5-6 pounds in squats and deadlifts, 4 pounds in your major upper body pressing movement, *and* 4 pounds in your major upper body pulling movement, *while maintaining the same form and number of repetitions.*

To add clarity, you will need to have increased all major movements as specified. If you only increase your bench press by 5 pounds, but none of the other movements improves by at least 5 pounds, you can't expect the pound of additional muscle, but perhaps only one-quarter pound or less. Increasing training loads in only one of the two major upper body movements means you have only added muscle to the groups responsible for performing that movement, not to the whole body, and that will have very little impact on your total body mass. You will get the largest increases in total body mass from progression in squats and deadlifts, so don't skip hard hip, thigh and back training if you want to gain muscle mass.

In the chin ups and dips, you will include your body weight in the total load for the exercise. For example, if you do 6 chin ups with a bodyweight of 155 and an additional load of 30 pounds, your total load is 185 pounds. If you progress to 6 chin ups at a bodyweight of 160 plus an external load of 45 pounds (205 pound total load), the total increase in load is 20 pounds with a body mass increase of 5 pounds. That's a 4:1 ratio of increased strength to increased body mass.

For more details about sustainable progressive resistance exercise, visit www.fullrangestrength.com or www.donmatesz.com.

If your body mass is going up without your training loads increasing at a faster rate, you are gaining more fat than muscle.

Meal timing around training

So long as your energy and protein intake is overall adequate to support muscle growth, the timing of the meals in relation to training is of secondary importance. The key dietary step is to eat a large, protein- and energy-rich meal within 3-4 hours on either side (before or after) doing your strength training.

This meal should contain at least 20 g protein if you are less than 40 years of age, and at least 40 g of protein if you are more than 40 years of age (elders show a blunted response to only 20 g protein).[108] If you train in the morning on an empty stomach, eat your meal within a few hours of finishing training. If you train in the evening, have the meal either a few hours before or shortly after the training session.

If you complete your training session within 3-4 hours of an adequate previous meal, there is a lack of evidence that eating immediately after a training

---

[108] Aragon A, Schoenfeld BJ, "Nutrient timing revisited: is there a post-exercise anabolic window?," *J Int Soc Sports Nutr* 2013 Jan 29;10:5 <https://jissn.biomedcentral.com/articles/10.1186/1550-2783-10-5>

session is necessary to obtain maximum gains.[109] Thus, if you eat morning and midday meals, you can train before breakfast, between the two meals, or 3-4 hours after the second meal, and in the latter case, do not need to take a post-training meal because nutrients available from the pre-training meal will be sufficient.

If you cannot start training until 5-6 hours after the midday meal, simply increase the energy and protein content of the midday meal; larger meals take longer to digest and create a longer post-meal anabolic window. If instead you eat a midday and evening meal, again you can train before the breakfast, between the two meals, or after the evening meal.

Eating for muscle gains

If you are already lean, you should train hard on a strength program and eat enough to satisfy the increase in hunger you will experience after training sessions. If you are not already in the lean category, you can maintain energy balance or deficit. If you can

---

[109] Ibid.

arrange your schedule for the purpose, you can take advantage of the anabolic effect of training by slightly increasing your food intake in the meal you consume before or after your training sessions.

Table 11.4: Example of a Possible Caloric Cycling Schedule to Promote Muscle Gains (assuming 2500 kcal maintenance requirements)	
Day	Caloric Intake
1 Resistance Training	3000
2	2600
3 Resistance Training	3000
4	2600
5 Resistance Training	3000
6	2600
7	2500

For example, let's say you need 2500 kcal daily to support your activities of daily living, and you expend 350 kcal in 1 hour of resistance training on Monday, Wednesday, and Friday mornings. After training you will feel increased hunger, and to satisfy this you eat 3000 kcal in your 6-8 hour feeding window. On your rest days – Tuesday, Thursday and Saturday – you might have a slightly increased hunger and consume 2600, and on Sunday you might have your baseline hunger level and consume only 2500 kcal. On Monday you start the cycle over. These numbers are hypothetical. This calorie-cycling program is depicted in Table 11.4.

Over the seven days, you will have spontaneously eaten a total of 1800 kcal above your baseline intake. Of this, 1050 covered the additional energy expended in training, so the remainder of 750 went to support muscle recovery and growth. Since a pound of muscle contains about 550 kcal, you probably have consumed enough to support the addition of at least one pound of muscle without force feeding yourself. In addition, you have eaten more primarily on the days you trained, ensuring that the additional food would go primarily to the promotion of lean weight gain, rather than fat stores; and you have fasted 16-20 hours on all days. You get all the health benefits of longer fasting periods, while also eating exactly what you needed – as dictated by your hunger – to support lean weight gain.

I have offered this hypothetical scenario just to show you that if you train yourself to trust your true Nature and follow its guidance, you do not have to force feed yourself to gain muscle. You are unique, and your training might make you want more or less food than I have suggested for my hypothetical scenario. Regardless, Nature provides you with the sense of hunger and it will not mislead you; you can and should rely upon it to guide you to consume exactly what you need, when you need it. In that way you can gain muscle without unnecessarily adding fat.

Hard, progressive training will increase your hunger. If you don't have increased hunger after training, don't force yourself to eat more. If your training does not increase your appetite, probably you have not yet reached a level of difficulty in your squats or deadlifts to produce a demand for more food. Check your training, and keep increasing the resistance incrementally; eventually your body will need to add some muscle and then you will want to eat more.

Pay special attention if you find yourself waking up hungry in the middle of the night. If this occurs, probably your training has stimulated gains, but you have failed to eat enough during the day. If you have unsatisfied hunger, and you aren't gaining 1-2 pounds per month, you haven't eaten enough: pay closer attention to your hunger and slightly increase your food intake on training days. Make sure you feel fully satisfied at the end of meals and end of your feeding window.

If your training stimulates the growth of about 1 pound of muscle per week, on some days you might need to consume about 400-800 additional kcalories in your feeding window. One easy way to do this without feeling stuffed and losing your appetite would be to maintain your normal size meals, but add whole milk or whole milk yogurt, either alone or blended with raw eggs – to be consumed in the few hours after your training session. Liquids are generally less satiating than solid food, making them ideal for adding energy to the diet without making you so full that it impairs your appetite for your regular meals. A cup of whole milk or whole milk yoghurt provides 150 calories, 8 g protein, 8 g fat, and 12 g carbohydrate. Two large whole eggs provide 155 kcal, 12 g protein, 10 g fat, and 1 g carbohydrate. A quart of whole milk or whole milk yoghurt will provide 600 kcal, 32 g protein, 32 g fat, and 48 g carbohydrate. You can reduce the carbohydrate by blending 2 cups milk or yoghurt with 4 eggs, which will provide 610 kcal, 28 g protein, 26 g fat, and 24 g carbohydrate.

If after adding liquid calories to your diet for a month or two you notice significant fat gain, you can conclude that you have been eating more than your hunger called for, or more carbohydrate than you can tolerate, or both. You may want to reduce the carbohydrate or caloric content unless you were too lean to begin with and needed to gain that fat.

To reiterate, one should focus on hard, progressive training, and if you do that you can generally let your appetite guide your food intake, because hard training that makes a demand for new muscle will generally increase your appetite a bit. Eat more only if you are hungry for more, not if you're not. If you're not hungry, your training is not hard or progressive enough to create a need for muscle growth.

Gaining muscle may be inhibited by continuous overeating and simultaneous gaining of fat tissue, but is supported by efficient assimilation and use of nutrients, and by reducing insulin resistance and myostatin expression. Since fasting improves digestive efficiency and improves insulin sensitivity, time-restricted feeding and primal fasting (and a high protein high fat diet) can help you gain muscle without gaining unwanted fat, provided you train hard and progressively over a long period of time.

12 Breaking Fast: Primal Feeding

Contrary to popular belief, brief fasting (16-36 hours) does not weaken the digestive system or make it necessary to only gradually reintroduce solid foods. On the contrary, after a fast of this length, you will have a strong appetite (a sign of a strong digestive system) and prefer and require substantial foods. Breaking a fast with a puny meal will only leave you unsatisfied.

Make sure your break-fast meals are substantial and nutrient-dense. Meat, eggs, fish, dairy products and animal fats are the best foods to consume post-fasting, as they provide sufficient energy and nutrient density to quickly satisfy your post-fast appetite without containing excessive carbohydrates that will wipe out the fat-burning benefits of the fasting.

Do you need carbohydrate in your breakfast? No. As previously mentioned, you have no dietary requirement for carbohydrate provided you consume adequate protein and fat.[110] Eating carbohydrate stimulates the release of insulin, and rapidly fills glycogen stores, both of which reduce utilization of fat for energy. The body can produce what glucose you need to form essential glycogen stores (as an emergency energy supply) from some amino acids and from the glycerol present in fats.

Calorie restriction, high intensity exercise (resistance training, sprinting) and very low carbohydrate diets produce a metabolic condition similar to but not as pronounced as fasting.[111, 112] Thus, combining high intensity exercise (resistance training) and a low carbohydrate diet with time-restricted feeding and

---

[110] Food and Nutrition Board, National Academy of Sciences. Dietary Reference Intakes for Energy, Carbohydrate, Fiber, Fat, Fatty Acids, Cholesterol, Protein, and Amino Acids. National Academies Press, 2005. Pages 275-6. "The lower limit of dietary carbohydrate compatible with life apparently is zero, provided that adequate amounts of protein and fat are consumed." <https://www.nap.edu/read/10490/chapter/8?term=carbohydrate+requirement#275>

[111] Ibid.

[112] Westman EC, Feinman RD, Mavropoulos JC, et al. Low-carbohydrate nutrition and metabolism. Am J Clin Nutr 2007 Aug; 86(2):276-84. <http://ajcn.nutrition.org/content/86/2/276.full>

intermittent fasting supports elevated ketone production for all the benefits discussed in chapter 7.

You can gain benefits from fasting regardless of your background diet, but I favor a primarily or completely carnivorous ancestral diet. All ancient *human* ancestors were hunters who, whenever possible, lived exclusively or largely on animal products consisting of animal flesh, organs, eggs and fats.[113, 114, 115, 116] Across cultures, people prefer eating animal protein and fat to eating plant foods.[117] Unlike natural plantivores and like other natural carnivores, our digestive system can not extract substantial amounts of energy from fiber,

---

[113] Meaning ancestors belonging to the human (*Homo*) genus.

[114] McKie R. Humans hunted for meat 2 million years ago. Anthropology, The Observer, The Guardian 2012 Sep 22. <https://www.theguardian.com/science/2012/sep/23/human-hunting-evolution-2million-years>

[115] Holzman D. Meat eating is an old human habit. New Scientist 2003 Sep 7. <https://www.newscientist.com/article/dn4122-meat-eating-is-an-old-human-habit/>

[116] Cordain L, Miller JB, Eaton SB, Mann N, Holt SHA, Speth JD. Plant-animal subsistence ratios and macronutrient energy estimations in worldwide hunter-gatherer diets. *Am J Clin Nutr* 2000;71:682-92.

[117] Abrams HL. The Preference for Animal Protein and Fat: A Cross-Cultural Survey. In: Harris M and Ross EB, eds. *Food and Evolution*. Philadelphia, PA: Temple University Press, 1987: 207.

the primary constituent of plants. In short, we are by nature carnivores. An ancestral diet makes fresh animal products the primary foods.

As mammals, humans by Nature rely on milk when infants. Because evolution conserves what works, milk from various animals contains the same basic constituents – types of protein, fat and carbohydrate, as well as vitamins and minerals – and only differ in proportions of these constituents. Hence, humans in general have a Natural pre-adaptation to consuming milk, even of non-human species. However, individuals vary in their retention of the juvenile ability to efficiently digest milk sugar and protein as they age (retention of juvenile characteristics is called neoteny). Those of us whose ancestors consumed milk products for millennia generally have little or no problem consuming dairy products in some amount. Those of us whose ancestors did not use dairy products as staple foods are more likely to have some dairy intolerance. Some of these people have no problem digesting raw (unpasteurized) milk, or fermented milk products (fermentation pre-digests or in the case of aged cheeses virtually eliminates the milk sugar). Many

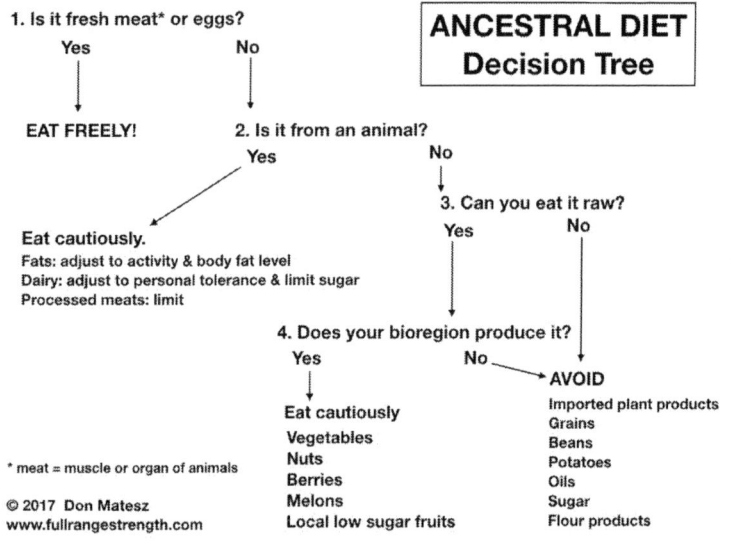

1. Is it fresh meat* or eggs?

Yes   No

ANCESTRAL DIET
Decision Tree

EAT FREELY!   2. Is it from an animal?

Yes   No

3. Can you eat it raw?

Yes   No

Eat cautiously.
Fats: adjust to activity & body fat level
Dairy: adjust to personal tolerance & limit sugar
Processed meats: limit

4. Does your bioregion produce it?

Yes   No ⟶ AVOID

* meat = muscle or organ of animals

© 2017 Don Matesz
www.fullrangestrength.com

Eat cautiously
Vegetables
Nuts
Berries
Melons
Local low sugar fruits

Imported plant products
Grains
Beans
Potatoes
Oils
Sugar
Flour products

people tolerate cream and cream products (butter, cream cheese) regardless of ancestry because cream has very little lactose or milk protein. Consequently, each individual must evaluate his/her own tolerance for various dairy products. You may want to cautiously experiment to determine which if any dairy products have no ill effect in your case, and how much of any type of dairy product you can consume beneficially.

By Nature, humans can consume and digest some raw plant foods, particularly fleshy fruits and berries, and soft greens. However, individual tolerance for these foods varies, possibly because our ancestors did not rely on plant foods but were highly carnivorous. You may consume some plant foods if you find you tolerate them, however you do not have to consume them. If you consume them at all, you should eat them cautiously, in modest amounts dictated by seasonal availability, and monitor your gut reaction, mental acuity and energy, and avoid or limit if you experience any adverse effects.

Plant products to consume cautiously include:
- Locally grown berries, melons and fruits
- Green and other non-starchy vegetables

Generally, because we have no enzymes for digestion of fiber, and vegetables are composed primarily of fiber, most people will find non-starchy vegetables more digestible and less harmful when pickled or cooked.

An ancestral diet limits or excludes plant foods that are either mostly indigestible and toxic in their natural (raw) state, or not found in Nature absent human interference. Those to include in only limited amounts include:

- most low-starch roots (e.g. beets, carrots)
- most nuts and seeds

Those to exclude or consume only on occasion (because of their high starch or toxin contents) include:

- starchy roots and tubers (e.g. potatoes, yams)
- mature dry cereal grains
- mature legumes (beans, peas, lentils)
- refined starches, sugars and proteins
- most oils derived from plants
- alcoholic beverages

These foods are harmful in several ways. They all have a low nutrient density and yet increase requirements for micronutrients. Except for berries and fruits, all plant parts, especially nuts, seeds, whole grains, legumes, and tubers contain some toxins that the plants make to discourage predators from consuming them.

Cereal grains and legumes contain a large amount of carbohydrate (sugar), and types of carbohydrate that promote metabolic disorders and gut inflammation. They also contain anti-nutrients such as phytate that block absorption of proteins, vitamins, and minerals.[118] Legumes are so toxic when raw or undercooked that eating some raw legumes can be fatal, and eating undercooked legumes can cause severe gut disorders.[119]

Starchy tubers contain a large amount of easily digested carbohydrate that stimulate spikes in blood glucose and insulin levels.[120] In addition they contain potential toxins. For example, common white potatoes contain about 8 mg solanine per 100 g potato, mostly in the skin. Since the toxic dose of solanine is 20-25 mg, eating 3 medium potatoes or one jumbo baking potato (with skin) can cause acute poisoning (vomiting, diarrhoea, abdominal pain).[121]

---

[118] Cordain L. Cereal Grains: Humanity's Double Edged Sword. *World Rev Nutr Diet* 1999;84:19-73.

[119] Freed DLJ. Editorial: Do dietary lectins cause disease? *BMJ* 1999 April 17;318:1023-1024.

[120] Bell K. Clinical Application of the Food Insulin Index to Diabetes Mellitus. Doctoral Thesis, University of Sydney 2014 Sep 5. <https://ses.library.usyd.edu.au/handle/2123/11945>

[121] US FDA. FDA Poisonous Plant Database. <https://www.accessdata.fda.gov/scripts/plantox/detail.cfm?id=1364>

Most plant-based oils contain high concentrations of the omega-6 fatty acid called linoleic acid. A basic principle of toxicology is: The dose makes the poison. The small amounts naturally present in unprocessed foods apparently do not have any harmful effects, but when extracted from foods and concentrated in free oils and consumed liberally (instead of natural animal fats) these fats appear to have multiple harmful effects, such as making skin more fragile and prone to sun damage, promoting inflammation, and promoting cancer.[122, 123, 124]

Alcohol is toxic. Consumption of alcohol weakens the will and impairs judgment, making one susceptible to doing stupid things or being controlled or misled by others. Alcohol may have been the first drug promoted by politicians to make others easier to manipulate and

[122] Ravnskov U. Myth 7: Polyunsaturated Oils are Good For You. In: The Cholesterol Myths: Exposing the Fallacy that Saturated Fat and Cholesterol Cause Heart Disease. Washington D.C.: New Trends Publishing Inc., 2000:217-234.

[123]Braden LM, Carroll KK. Dietary polyunsaturated fat in relation to mammary carcinogenesis in rats. *Lipids* 1986; 21:285-88.

[124] Toborek M, Lee YW, Garrido R, Kaiser S, Hennig B. Unsaturated fatty acids selectively induce an inflammatory environment in human endothelial cells. *Am J Clin Nutr* 2002; 75:119-125.

to lure them into agriculture and civilization.[125] As previously noted, the Roman historian Tacitus observed how alcohol undermined the native Germans:

> "A liquor for drinking is made out of barley or other grain, and fermented into a certain resemblance to wine. The dwellers on the river-bank also buy wine...They satisfy their hunger without elaborate preparation and without delicacies. In quenching their thirst they are not equally moderate. If you indulge their love of drinking by supplying them with as much as they desire, they will be overcome by their own vices as easily as by the arms of an enemy."[126]

Did the Romans conquer Germany because Germans habitually drank themselves into a stupor? Power-hungry politicians always exploit the weaknesses of their prey. They encourage addiction to stupefying drugs and circuses that will keep the people from becoming aware of the politicians' plans for power expansion. Beware, if you habitually impair your

---

[125] Wadley G, Hayden B. Pharmacological Influences on the Neolithic Transition. J Ethnobio 35(3):566-84.

[126] Tacitus. Germania and Agricola. Ostara Publications, 2016. Page 9-10.

awareness with alcohol or any other drug, you may not know what's up until its too late for you to do anything about it, and end up enslaved to sober invaders, the way the Germans ended up as subjects of Rome.

Alcohol promotes obesity because metabolism of alcohol almost completely stops the body from using fat as a fuel. It also destroys brain and liver cells. Although people have been led to believe that "moderate" alcohol consumption helps to prevent cardiovascular disease, a 1998 review found that the evidence for a cardio-protective effect for alcohol is weak.[127] Even if we grant alcohol the benefit of doubt, the cardiovascular advantage is insignificant and only associated with very small doses, 10 to 20 grams of alcohol—3 to 4 ounces of wine daily. Larger amounts are linked to more damage than benefit.[128] In France, where chronic alcohol consumption is claimed to play a role in protection from cardiovascular disease, the

---

[127] Svardsudd K. Moderate alcohol consumption and cardiovascular disease: is there evidence for a preventive effect? *Alcohol Clin Exp Res* (United States)1998 Oct. 22(7 Suppl): 307S-314S.

[128] Sasaki S. Alcohol and its relation to all-cause and cardiovascular mortality. *Acta Cardiol* (Belgium) 2000 Jun.;55(3): 151-6

death rate from liver cirrhosis increased by 163 percent overall (208 percent for French men and 186 percent for French women) between 1925 and 1982.[129]

---

[129] Coppere H, Audigier JC. Trends of mortality from cirrhosis in France between 1925 and 1982. *Gastroenterol Clin Biol* (France) 1986 Jun-Jul;10(6-7):468-74.

Additional Reading

Berkhan M. www.leangains.com

Johnson JB, Laub DR. The Alternate-Day Diet: Turn on Your "Skinny Gene," Shed the Pounds, and Live a Longer and Healthier Life. Perigree Books, 2009.

Pilon B. Eat Stop Eat. Strength Works, Inc., 2010.

Pilon B. How Much Protein? Strength Works, Inc., 2008-2009.

Matesz T. The Trust Your True Nature Low Carb Diet Plan. CreateSpace, 2018.

Mattson MP, Allison DB, Fontana L, et al. Meal frequency and timing in health and disease. Proceedings of the National Academy of Sciences of the United States of America. 2014;111(47): 16647-16653. doi:10.1073/pnas.1413965111.

Trepanowski JF, Bloomer RJ. The impact of religious fasting on human health. Nutrition Journal. 2010;9:57. doi:10.1186/1475-2891-9-57.

33114598R00081

Printed in Great Britain
by Amazon